The Diet

The Diet

◆

The Diet to Lose Weight and Feel Healthy!

30 days to a New Diet Life Style
Vegetarian and Omnivore Friendly

Brady Barrows

iUniverse, Inc.
New York Lincoln Shanghai

The Diet
The Diet to Lose Weight and Feel Healthy!

iUniverse, Inc.

For information address:
iUniverse, Inc.
2021 Pine Lake Road, Suite 100
Lincoln, NE 68512
www.iuniverse.com

Legal Disclaimer

The information contained in this book is not meant to substitute for medical care or treatment. You should consult with your doctor, health care provider, or nutritionist before changing your current diet.

www.the-diet-book.com

ISBN: 0-595-28996-7

Printed in the United States of America

To those who want a new diet life style…

diet *noun.* the food and drink normally taken by an individual or a group, *a diet of bread and cheese, a balanced diet* || a prescribed course of what is to be eaten and what is not

diet *verb transitive.* to put on a diet || *verb intransitive.* to eat special food (for health reasons, athletic training etc.) || to eat less so as to become thinner

life style 2. The way in which an individual lives, e.g., as to dress, habits, friendships, values, etc.

New Webster's Dictionary and Thesaurus of the English Language, 1993, Lexicon Publications, Inc. Danbury, CT.

Contents

Preface

In 1999 I began writing a diet to control rosacea which culminated in a paperback book published in the year 2002 by iUniverse which proved to be effective in helping rosaceans control their rosacea. Users of the *Rosacea Diet* reported losing weight and feeling healthier. The feedback (grin:) from this group inspired me to write this book for a much *larger* audience who want to lose weight or feel healthier.

Have you heard of 'elimination' diets, whatever that term implies? I suppose, depending on your definition of an elimination diet, the 30 Day Diet Plan for Meat Eaters and the 30 Day Diet Plan for Vegetarians in this book might be classified as an elimination diet by some. Possibly those who use the term 'elimination' diet in a disparaging and high brow manner to browbeat diets, so I don't use this term to describe *The Diet*. What I prefer is to describe *The Diet* as a life style change. If you accept the definition in the epigraph of this book that describes the noun, diet, as "a prescribed course of what is to be eaten and what is not" this book is simply a diet. You should think of this as *the diet*.

Acknowledgements

The following are acknowledged for their insight on diet for which I am grateful:

William Dufty, Sidney W. Mintz, Michael R. Eades, M.D., Mary Dan Eades, M.D., H. Leighton Steward, Morrison C. Bethea, M.D., Sam S. Andrews, M.D., Luis A. Balart, M.D., Robert C. Atkins, M.D., Carol Ann Rinzler, and Nicholas V. Perricone, M.D.

And a special thanks to Joyce Demarzi who proofread, critiqued and challenged me.

Introduction

In the twenty-first century obesity plagues the planet while at the same time millions are malnurished and hungry. What a sad paradox...

The Diet Authority

You have heard of the two most controversial subjects—religion and politics, right? There is a third, diet. You don't think so? These three subjects have been debated as far back as the Garden of Eden when a diet involved religion and sovereignty. You don't think diet is controversial? Why are there so many diet books? Try discussing diet with your friends, family or strangers and note the reaction. Everyone is a *diet authority*. Everyone knows what *you* should eat or what *you* shouldn't eat. Discussing what to eat and drink involves human emotion. Ask a vegetarian to explain tofu to a meat eater. Have fun storming the castle!

The big question is, 'what is the *correct* diet? Yes, what is *The Diet*? And who is to say what is the correct diet? By what authority does any person or organization have to say what is the correct diet? Even if the highest authority you can think of told you what to eat and drink, would you follow the diet suggested? Adam and Eve had a problem with the *diet authority*. Most people ignore the 'correct diet' since everyone wants to make their own decision as to what to eat and drink. And choosing what to eat and drink is a basic human right so universally accepted that it is not in any Bill of Rights or Universal Declaration of Human Rights. It is simply understood by everyone that an adult can choose whatever he or she wants to eat and drink without impunity or restrictions.

An example of a people who ignore a *diet authority* is in the USA. Most Americans who eat the 'average American diet' have largely ignored the USDA's Food Guide Pyramid created in 1992. *Newsweek*[1] magazine describes this diet as "…with a cherry on top. Sweets and meats are a bigger draw than healthful fruits and vegetables." No one likes a food cop. What if the government forced everyone to eat the Food Guide Pyramid or some other *authorized* diet? Diet should be added to the list following religion and politics as the third most controversial subject. This book will add to the controversy because I have no initials behind

---

1.   *Newsweek*, January 20, 2003, p.52

my name, like M.D., Ph.D., or whatever. I am not a nutritionist. I am simply an average American who discovered what helps to lose weight and feel healthier. There are thousands of diet books—the sheer number of them proves there is controversy. The more popular the diet book is the more controversy it brings. The browbeating, mud slinging, and criticism against and among diet book writers, critics, and diet authorities are cornucopian.

Michael Fumento has a website[2] discussing this controversy and wrote an interesting article entitled, *Living Off the Fat Only People Benefiting From Diet Books are the Authors* (*Washington Monthly*, Jan–Feb 18). In this article he wrote about the first diet guru, appearing more than a century ago, William Banting, who actually got his diet from the British ear surgeon William Harvey. Banting lost weight on this diet and later published the diet as *Banting's Letter on Corpulence*. Since Banting's background wasn't in health, but rather he was an undertaker, this established the precedent that anyone can write a diet book. My book is based on research and the success of my first book, the *Rosacea Diet*, and the user feedback over a period of four years. I am basically self-taught and learned most of my nutrition on health from Carol Ann Rinzler's book[3] and other books I mention. I was an EMT for about ten years but that doesn't even get me a cup of coffee. My certification expired years ago.

My belief is that wisdom is proved righteous by its works. *The Diet* works. You will decide for yourself. That is what this chapter is about. Do you think that thirty-days on my diet poses any health risks? No. It is important that you understand that this diet is for thirty days. After that you decide what you want to do with this diet.

The Diet is a way of thinking and a lifestyle. Who is the authority to tell you what to eat and drink? Am I? You have got to be kidding. I can't convince you what to eat and drink. Only you can decide this for yourself, since it a basic human right understood universally that you decide what to eat and drink for yourself.

So why would you bother to read a book telling you what to eat and drink? Information. You obviously want information. So what makes this book *The Diet*? So far I haven't found a diet book with that title and it should work good as a keyword in any search engine ☺. I am confident that *the diet* can change the way

---

2.   http://www.fumento.com
3.   *Nutrition for Dummies*, Carol Ann Rinzler, 1997, IDG Books Worldwide, Inc.

you think about food and drink and will help you control your weight and feel healthier.

You will hear about 30 days, 30 grams and many other things repetitively. I learned over the past few years that when people read my first book they asked me repetitive questions so my reaction is to follow the same pattern and be repetitive in my writing to prevent frequently asked questions.

Why would you want to change your diet? You are already on a diet according to the dictionary definition mentioned in the epigraph of this book. There are only two reasons possible I can think of—(1) to lose weight or (2) to feel healthier. I challenge you to come up with another reason. You may not have given much thought about why you eat the way you do, but you obviously are thinking about it now. Stop and think for a moment about your current diet. Your mother (or whoever fed you in childhood) made choices you make now. You trusted Mom (or whoever fed you) and so how can Mom be wrong about diet? This is not to say that Mom did not have your best interest at heart. The point is that you probably were influenced to choose the food and drink that is on your current diet and this also has an emotional impact on your life. Food is such a controversial subject since what we eat and drink has an emotional impact on our lives. Food and drink should impact our emotional state for the better. At a party the food and drink can play such an important emotional impact on the event as to whether it is successful or not. Whatever emotional state we are in, whether happy, sad, or under stress, food has such a tremendous emotional impact on us. Try eating or drinking with an enemy of yours? The way we respond to life stresses is so deeply psychologically rooted in us that sometimes we don't realize what we are doing to ourselves. Remember the saying, *you are what you eat*? You are also what your mom gave you to eat. Mom learned how to eat and drink from her mother and so on. So what is the point? The authority that first influenced you to eat was Mom or you may have been impacted by another *diet authority* or diet book. Is it possible that Mom has been wrong about diet? Could your Mom have been influenced to give you food that isn't healthy for you? How could Mom be wrong? How can there be so many diet books with so many different approaches from so many different *diet authorities* especially when you consider there are only three basic food groups and every diet just juggles the three around? Why is there so much controversy?

It has been said that, "uncertainties still cloud our understanding of the relation between diet and health[4]." Yet we know there is a relationship between diet and health. So lets take a history lesson with food, a lesson you haven't thought about till now. The human race has not been eating and drinking the same way since the beginning. A change started to occur around 1700, the beginning of the eighteenth century. What am I talking about?

For millenniums mankind generally ate fruit, vegetables, dairy, eggs, grains, seafood, fish, fowl, and meats. Anthropologically speaking, a big change in diet started to occur just a few hundred years ago resulting in a dramatic change in diet that has effected the choices you and your Mom are making in food and drink. This change effected *diet authorities* in the Twentieth Century and dramatically changed the diet mankind eats today. Diet books and *diet authorities* have been impacted by what happened. What happened? The sugar industry began to emerge with great economic power. I have arbitrarily chosen the beginning of the Eighteenth Century as the start of the *'Sugar Age'* since statistics show that the average Englishman ate 4 pounds of sugar a year at this point and before this very little consumption of sugar is known.

Later the sugar industry became part of the processed food industry of the twentieth century. The processed food industry has a tremendous impact on a major portion of the planet economically thus effecting your choice of food and drink especially with the advent of globalization. This is not to say that the processed food industry is intrinsically bad. Certainly having food and drink processed has many advantages. It is nice to see food protected in clear plastic wrap. Having safe food and drink clean and free from contaminates is wonderful. Having food processed makes obtaining it easier and quicker for billions of people. The main advantage usually is that the price of food processed by an industry is cheaper than food we could grow ourselves, not to mention the convenience. Besides, in this system who has the time or ability to grow or raise their own food? There are no doubt other good things to say about the processed food industry. But the choice you make as to what you eat and drink is certainly influenced by this industry probably more than you may have thought. Could there be something in the processed food industry that may be causing obesity or other health problems? How much influence do you think the processed food industry has on you or your Mom?

---

4. *Scientific American*, January 2003, Rebuilding the Food Guide Pyramid, Walter C. Willett and Meir J. Stampfer

Since the last century the *'diet authorities'* have pointed to **fat** as the culprit[5] for health problems. Hence, a plethora of fat free or low fat diets and products have been offered, and the processed food industry responded with low fat (or without fat) food and drink. The advertising of these products influences millions, if not billions. Yet when you look at the results over the last century obesity has risen particularly since 1992. In the developed world obese people are at a record high despite what the *'diet authorities'* have said about the dangers of eating too much fat. A Worldwatch Institute study reveals that the overfed now equals the underfed. Some 1.2 billion people are underfed and hungry and an equal number or more now eat too much. *The New York Times* commented on this study by saying,

> "The number of overweight people in the world now rivals the number of hungry, underfed people."

The Worldwatch Institute's *State of the World 2000* states,

> "Half the world's people, both rich and poor, are medically malnourished, suffering from either obesity or from diets with inadequate calories, vitamins, or minerals. A whopping 55 percent of American adults are overweight."

This paradox doesn't make any sense. As the processed food industry of the developed world makes inroads into the underdeveloped world the result is a diet producing obesity. What does the underdeveloped people of the world die of? Primarily the cause of death is infectious diseases due to malnutrition and poor hygiene. What is the primary cause of death in the developed world? The cause is primarily what the World Health Organization classifies as "Noncommunicable Conditions" which include vascular disorders (such as heart disease, stroke and diabetes) and all cancers. Diet is a factor in these deaths. What accounts for the obesity in the developed world? While fat has been the accused culprit in the minds of many, there is another culprit emerging as the culprit, *sugar*.

A growing number of people have discovered that sugar is the cause of obesity. How is this possible? Simply, excess sugar in the diet is converted to fat. It is an undisputed fact that sugar is a factor in obesity. The processed food industry uses

---

5.   "The belief that fat is the dietary bad guy is about as close to universal as any idea in America."—*The World's Biggest Fad Diet* by Dean Esmay source > http://www. survivediabetes.com/lowfat.html

sugar in a large percentage of the food and drink prepared and sold to the world. Most people in the world are ignorant of this or don't care. Historically sugar's health problems have either been minimized or dismissed by the *'diet authorities'* and the processed food industry. Coupled with the fast food industry which also uses sugar in its food and drink the results are that 55% of American adults are overweight and the rest of the developed world is trying to catch up to the Americans in obesity. Some figures indicate that the number of obese Americans is even higher. As the processed food industry moves into underdeveloped countries obesity rises and along with it rises in vascular disorders and cancers which shows the influence this industry has on people's choices.

Why is sugar used in such large percentages in the processed food industry? Basically it is cheap to produce, yields higher profit, makes the food taste better, and is addictive. As Sidney W. Mintz writes in his book, *Sweetness and Power—The Place of Sugar in Modern History*, on page 190–191,

> "Per hectare (2.7 acres), sugar cane yields, under optimum conditions, about twenty tons of dry material, some half of which is in the form of sugar usable as food or feed; the other ten tons of cane 'trash,' or bagasse, is usable as fuel and for the manufacture of paper products, building materials, and furfuraldehyde (a liquid aldehyde used in manufacturing nylon and resins, and as a solvent)…An acre of good subtropical land will now produce more than eight million calories in sugar, beyond the other products it yields…antisaccarites are compelled to recognize sugar's appeal on grounds of taste, energy economy, relative cost, and calories—an appeal sugar manufacturers clearly recognize, and which their political, professorial, and professional supporters push vigorously."

Professor Mintz writes on page 192,

> "Where the need for calories, let alone other food values, is a serious problem, sucrose may not be a good nutritional answer (in large quantities, I think it is a terrible one); but circumstances early made it, and have kept it, what looks like a good economic answer. When one adds to this the remarkable energy-transforming nature of plants like sugar cane and maize—even at high levels of human input in the form of fertilizers, cultivation, etc., the solar-energy input is approximately 0 percent of the total energy consumed in producing a usable food—the appeal of sucrose as a solution to food problems becomes almost irresistible."

Professor Mintz's book is a remarkable anthropological insight into the power of the sugar industry and the change sugar has made on mankind in the relatively short period of just the last few centuries. Westernization, modernization, industrialization, globalization or the modern development of the world cannot be fully understood historically or anthropologically without sucrose power as a factor to consider. The power of the sugar industry is tremendous. Most sugar in the world has traditionally or historically! been the sucrose from sugar cane or sugar beets. Now high fructose corn syrup (HFCS) has exceeded the production of sugar cane or sugar beet sucrose. This billion-dollar sugar industry whether made from sucrose or high fructose corn syrup has had tremendous impact on your diet. Can you imagine the economic impact a company like Coca-Cola ® has on mankind in selling its product? That is just one company pushing sugar not only in the developed world but now in practically every country of the underdeveloped world. And does Coke ® know how to sell its product? Is it successful? A thirsty, sugar-loving people of the world love Coke ® because of the advertising and promotion of this product, not to mention its wonderful taste[6]. I am simply using this example to help you see the impact of the economic power of sugar. So many major corporations use sugar or high fructose corn syrup. When *Coca-Cola* ® changed from sucrose to high fructose corn syrup this had a major impact why HFCS has now become the largest sugar processed and consumed.

So your choices as to food and drink have been impacted to a large degree to eat sugar in greater quantities. At the turn of the Eighteenth Century (1700) the average Englishman ate four (4) pounds of sugar a year. By the turn of the Nineteenth Century (1800) it had risen to 18 pounds a year (*Sweetness and Power*, page 67). However, the United States by 1880-8 was consuming 38 pounds of sucrose per person per year, the second highest consumer just under the British (Sweetness and Power, page 188). When the Twentieth Century rolled around the British and the Americans were neck and neck since the per-capita figure for the first time rose above 90 pounds per person. (*Sweetness and Power*, page 143) From then till 1996 the figures keep rising to 149 pounds[7] per person in the USA! These figures are similar in European countries with the English and the Icelandic the largest consumers of sugar in a world that competes to be in first place in sugar consumption. What this means is that the production and consumption of sugar has increased dramatically only in the last two to three hun-

6.   It would be nice if Diet Coke ® would use Stevia as a sugar substitute
7.   *Sugar Busters!* by H. Leighton Steward, Dr. Morrison C. Bethea, Dr. Samued Dr. Luis A Balart, 1995, *Sugar Busters!*, LLC, Figure 2, page 43

dred years! You and your Mom have been eating quite differently than your ancestors that lived before the *Sugar Age*.

An interesting tidbit is that at the beginning of the twentieth century most sugar consumed was purchased by itself and then used in food or drink. The consumer added sugar to what was consumed. By the end of the century most sugar consumed is now already added in food and drink processed. Since most people purchase small amounts of sugar by itself a consumer may be mislead into thinking that very little sugar is being consumed. However the facts show that the average consumer is eating tremendous amounts of sugar from processed food and drink.

While sucrose has historically been the main focus of the sugar industry, there is a growing industry of alternative sugars, such as high fructose corn syrup, sugar substitutes and other sugars. The list of sugars is massive (see the chapter *Sugars to Avoid*). High Fructose Corn Syrup (HFCS) has now reached greater production than sucrose made from either sugar cane or beets. Mintz writes on page 73 of his book that this consumption of sugar "may be enough to say that probably no other food in world history has had a comparable performance." Two exhaustive works on food[8] both give a significant amount of discussion on sugar and desserts. *The Cambridge World History of Food* by Kenneth F. Kiple & Kriemhild Conee Ornelee has been called the 'food book of the millennium' by *Science Magazine*. It states,

> "...for those seeking a "heart-healthy" diet...wonder that despite their increasing longevity, many people in the developed world have become abruptly and acutely anxious about what they do and do not put in their mouths...Nor are developing-world peoples so likely as those in the developed world to survive the nutritional disorders that seem to be legacies of our hunter-gatherer past. Diabetes (which may be the result of a "thrifty" gene for carbohydrate metabolism) is one of these diseases, and hypertension may be another; still others are doubtless concealed among a group of food allergies, sensitivities, and intolerances that have only recently begun to receive the attention they deserve..."

---

8. *The Cambridge World History of Food* by Kenneth F. Kiple & Kriemhild Conee Ornelee, Cambridge University Press > http://www.cup.org/books/kiple/default.htm
    The Oxford Companion to Food by Alan Davidson, Oxford University Press 1999

The above quote helps to understand everyone's concern about diet. You would think that nutritionists and medical authorities (*diet authorities*) would be in agreement on what the *perfect* diet should be. When you bring the processed food industry into the picture, economics becomes the factor in this disunity. The *diet authorities* are impacted by this industry. Capitalism, greed, emotions, nutrition and basic human rights are in a tangled mess when it comes to deciding what factors influence your choice of food and drink.

The *Newsweek* magazine article, *Stacking up the Perfect Diet*,[9] mentions "millions of Americans who desperately want to change their unhealthy ways, but can't quite get started." On page 6 of this magazine it states,

> "The federal government has long tried to distill the best science on diet and health. But commercial pressures and bureaucratic obstacles have often clouded the results. The USDA's famous Food Guide Pyramid, first published in 1992, is now widely viewed as flawed. 'The pyramid is a disaster,' says K. Dun Gifford of Oldways, a non-profit think tank based in Boston. 'The American epidemic of obesity is the proof that it hasn't worked. Period. Amen.'"

The economic pressure of the processed food industry on Americans, as well as on the rest of the world is summed up nicely on page 51 of this same magazine:

> "A second point of consensus is that vegetables should be eaten in abundance. There isn't a diet guru who denies their virtues. Heart doctors endorse them, cancer doctors endorse them, the USDA endorses them, and even the low-carb king Dr. Robert Atkins endorses them. Unfortunately, no one can afford to promote spinach or bell peppers the way snackmakers promote their goods. McDonald's spent $1.1 billion on advertising in 2001. That same year the budget for the governments' pro-vegetable '5 a Day for Better Health' program was 1.1 *million*. Not surprisingly, only 23 percent of U.S. adults were meeting the five-a-day target at last count."

Mom and the processed food industry have conditioned you to eat and drink the 'average American diet' and now you want to change your diet? When Mom gave you ice cream, apple pie and a *Coke* ® you felt happy and trusted Mom. She was giving you comfort. Now you want to change your diet? This is not going to be easy. You have to be motivated. Hopefully this book will be the motivating fac-

---

9.   *Newsweek*, January 20, 2003, p.44–5

tor. The motivation is short term to lose weight but in the long term for lifelong health.

Getting back to the question, 'Who is the Diet Authority?" **The diet authority is you**. You can read all the diet books on the planet for information or listen to the 'food cops' but you still decide what to eat and drink. As long as there is choice in the food and drink available, you are the *diet authority*. Maybe soylent green[10] will be all that is available but for now you have a choice. However, the emotional impact when Mom, a 'food cop,' a friend or the processed food industry offers you food or drink is very deep. You may react with feelings that are so deep rooted you need to come to grips with *WHO IS THE DIET AUTHORITY?*' **You are**.

---

10. *Soylent Green* (1973) is a film directed by Richard Fleischer based on a novel by Harry Harrison (Make Room! Make Room!) starring Charlton Heston, screenplay by Harry Harrison and Stanley R. Greenberg—if you haven't seen the film, I rate it a two star film worth watching. You will never forget it once you see it.

Protein and Fat—Essential for Life

Essential food and drink may be obvious to you but you may be surprised at the following statement. Protein, fat, and water are essential to life, but carbohydrates are not. If you were on a desert island or the moon you can survive on protein, fat and water. If you strictly only had carbohydrates you would eventually die. Why?

Carbohydrate is a word derived from Greek meaning 'carbon plus water.' All carbohydrates are composed of units of sugars and could be called the *dessert* of food. Carbohydrate is broken down to glucose, which is essential to human life. Glucose and oxygen is essential for cell survival and the fuel of the body. However, you can obtain glucose from protein and fat. You cannot get protein or fat from carbohydrates. It is impossible and an indisputable fact. You can obtain glucose from all three food groups, carbohydrates, protein and fat. But on a desert island if you only had carbohydrates you would die! For example, if the only food source was table sugar, a carbohydrate, and you even had water, eventually you would actually go bonkers and die[1]. You would die of malnutrition. You need protein and fat. Of course you also need certain vitamins, minerals, fiber, and a host of other things to survive, but I am trying to make a point about carbohydrate. Try to be open-minded and give me a break. My purpose in this chapter is to establish protein and fat as essential to life. I am on a roll here and you need to keep up.

---

1. *Sugar Blues*, William Dufty, 1975, Warner Books, Inc., describes in the chapter, *Dead Dogs and Englishman*, about a shipwrecked vessel in 1793 with five surviving sailors marooned for just nine days rescued in a wasted condition due to starvation. The sailors had subsisted on a diet of sugar and rum. As Dufty wrote on page 137, "Refined sugar is lethal when ingested by humans because it provides only that which nutritionists describe as empty or naked calories. In addition, sugar is worse than nothing because it drains and leeches the body of precious vitamins and minerals through the demand its digestion, detoxification, and elimination make upon one's entire system."

Most plants (vegetables, grains, fruits, nuts, etc.) contain mostly carbohydrate but may contain also some protein and fat. So when you eat plants you may obtain all three food groups. Fish, seafood, eggs, and meat contain protein and fat but usually no carbohydrate and in rare exceptions have trace amounts of carbohydrates. A three-ounce slice of beef liver, for instance, contains 22.4 grams of protein, 9 grams of fat, and 4.5 grams of carbohydrates. Who would ever think that liver has carbohydrate! Dairy may have all three food groups but in some cases zero carbohydrates. Cream has fat and protein but no carbohydrate!

The human health requirement for protein established by most reputable health authorities is between 50 to 100 grams a day depending on several factors such as age, weight, sex, activity, etc. If you are in a concentration camp the above requirement for protein will keep you alive, but probably not very healthy. You obviously need more than 50 to 100 grams of protein! But remember that if you fail to get protein you will die. If you don't get enough protein you will be unhealthy. Absolute fact. There is a debate among health professionals that you can eat too much protein. However this debate is foolish when you simply think of the Eskimo who at one time lived on a diet high in protein and fat, and some Eskimo may still eat this way! But the sad fact is that more and more Eskimo are drinking soft drinks and eating twinkies.

Think about overeating protein. Imagine the Eskimo overeating protein. Will the Eskimo die or be unhealthy? Are you going to tell the Eskimo to stop eating a high protein diet? Imagine a *diet authority* browbeating the high protein diet of the Eskimo or claiming that what the Eskimo ate is unhealthy or that he may have a disease creating a problem digesting protein? But these same health critics on diets will browbeat any high protein diet and site all sorts of reasons, shouting about the waste products created in high protein diets. These pale into insignificance when you mention the Eskimo. How did the Eskimo manage the waste products from eating a high protein diet and survive for all these millenniums? For that matter the Australian aborigine is another group to bring up. There are other groups or cultures eating a high protein, high fat diet and survived.

Lets discuss the usual warnings given for eating a high protein diet. People with certain diseases have problems processing protein, like gout, and so *diet authorities* browbeat high protein diets based on the possibility that a person might have a disease that impairs digesting protein, so therefore, according to this logic high protein diets are bad. Actually this is begging the question. The issue is whether eating a high protein diet is unhealthy, not whether a person has a problem digesting protein. The critics of high protein diets say eating a high protein diet may result in not being able to digest protein, which has never been proven. It is just a theory. Reasonably most people do not have diseases that would create a problem digesting protein and can eat as much protein as they want. The other issue is with waste products produced from eating a high protein diet that may produce health problems. Again, this is begging the question. The issue is whether eating a high protein diet is healthy, not the possibility of having a problem removing waste from a high protein diet. Most humans have no problem handling waste products from protein and there is no evidence that humans eating a high protein diet can not handle the waste products in the normal manner. The waste products from protein are simply eliminated from the body in the normal manner. Drs. Eades of *Protein Power* fame have explained in their books that eating a high protein diet is healthy and they are not the only medical doctors saying this. High protein diets are healthy even though the health critics lambaste those who endorse such diets. Remember the Eskimo.

Fat is required for human health and the health authorities have established the magic number of no more than thirty percent of your total daily calories[2] should be fat. On the Greek Island of Crete the traditional diet constitutes 40 percent fat of the total caloric intake. The rate of heart disease on this island is less than on the island of Japan, where the traditional diet is only 8 to 10 per cent fat. Imagine the *diet authorities* warning the inhabitants of Crete for eating too much fat.

Thirty percent of a 2,000-calorie diet would amount to 600 calories or 66.7 grams of fat. Fat has nine calories per gram. Fat is what nutritionists and health authorities call lipids. All lipids are divided into three groups, triglycerides, phospholipids, and sterols. All three are essential to life. If you are on that desert island you must obtain all three forms of fat or you die. That is a fact. The triglycerides are the fat composed of three essential fatty acids floating around in your blood that can be burned by the body cells for energy if needed. That is just one thing triglycerides are good for. If you don't have glucose in your blood, triglycerides may be used to burn energy by converting fatty acids into glucose. Amazing, isn't it? And you thought triglycerides are bad, didn't you? Who told you that? You need triglycerides.

---

2.   "The 30 percent limit on fat was essentially drawn from thin air."—Scientific American, January 2003, Rebuilding the Food Guide Pyramid, Walter C. Willett and Meir J. Stampfer

Fat is used in your cells as a membrane. Myelin, the fatty material that sheathes nerve cells, is composed of fat. These are just some examples of how you need fat. Can you eat too much fat and have problems? That is an unctuous subject. Think again of the Eskimo. How did the Eskimo survive on a diet high in fat and protein? They did it despite all the health warnings from the *diet authorities* that eating too much fat is unhealthy. The Australian aborigines in times past or present also ate a high fat and protein diet in the bush. Imagine the *diet authorities* criticizing their diet?

Fat is probably the most studied and talked about food of *diet authorities* and nutritionists. The alleged dangers of fat are notorious and swollen. Don't you just love puns? You can read all about saturated, unsaturated, monounsaturated, polyunsaturated, cholesterol, lipoproteins (HDLs and LDLs), triglycerides, etc., and get insulated in a fat discussion with your health care provider who no doubt has some very entrenched beliefs about fat. Just about everyone puts trans fats down which is no doubt a good idea. Just remember that all health authorities recommend you eat no more than 66.7 grams of fat or the magic number of thirty percent of your total caloric intake. Another big debate is that the red meat contains 'bad' fat while the 'good' fat is in plants, fish, and seafood. Stop and think of the American Indian who ate a diet high in the red meat of the buffalo and other game animals. Can you imagine a nutritionist putting down an American Indian eating all that fat from red meat?

It is universal that you can eat fat since just about every *diet authority* allows up to the magic number 30 per cent of the total caloric intake. The debate is over which fats and if you eat more than thirty per cent. But you can eat fat, which is my point! Fat is not the bad guy. We need fat, and fat is good! Fat really is the good guy! The mantra from the health authorities for the past thirty or more years that 'fat is bad' is no doubt deeply rooted in your heart. But take heart, you need fat!

Everyone needs cholesterol to survive which is fat. Cholesterol is in your cells, your organs, and glands. Cholesterol is essential for human health. It is used as the base for building steroid hormones such as estrogen and testosterone. Bile is made from cholesterol. We need cholesterol. Why has cholesterol been given such a bad reputation? There are many reasons but it isn't because you do not need cholesterol since you do. If you are on that desert island you must somehow obtain cholesterol or you die. You may have a problem with cholesterol but it is not because you don't need cholesterol! If you don't have cholesterol you die! I am repeating this because the health authorities have given cholesterol such a bad reputation that you may feel that your cholesterol level somehow is related to being a friend of Hitler. Your cholesterol level can bring you into some sort of panic attack because of all this worry over what it should be. Cholesterol is essential fat. So give cholesterol and fat a break. You deserve to eat your fat or your cholesterol without guilt and you can eat up to thirty per cent of fat in your diet!

Now one of the big debates is over the 'bad' cholesterol and sorting out the 'good' cholesterol. The 'bad' cholesterol is actually a misnomer since both are essential for human health. Again it is the amount and ratios that are debated and whether your high and low density lipoproteins are within the norms. But there is no debate over the fact that we need both types of high and low density lipoproteins. Actually you have been mislead by the *diet authorities* because in your mind the HDLs and LDLs are fat, but as the acronym points out they are protein particles carrying cholesterol. They are the same particle depending on whether the particle takes cholesterol into the blood vessels (LDLs) or carries it out of the body (HDLs). So much for your cholesterol lesson. Anyway, we need both for survival. 30 per cent fat is ok. 'Fat is good' should be your new mantra. Cholesterol is good too! Three cheers for triglycerides!!!

Now the final food group is carbohydrate. If you just had plenty of table sugar on that desert island (which is a carbohydrate) and plenty of water you would still die of malnutrition if that is all you had. The human health requirement for carbohydrate is zero[3]. That is a fact. *Diet authorities* have recommended a diet high in carbohydrate over the last century especially since 1992 when the USDA officially endorsed carbohydrates, a food group not essential for human health. Americans have high carbohydrated their life style ever since. Health and *diet authorities* have praised the carbohydrate to the maximum, a food group not essential for survival, and instead attacked fat, giving minimal praise to protein. In the minds of the typical American, the health authorities have established the mantra 'fat is bad' and 'carbohydrates are good.' Protein is minimized with barely an honorable mention giving you the idea that if you eat too much protein you will eat too much fat and you should worry about this.

However, a growing group of *diet authorities* have bravely published that a diet high in protein is healthy. This book joins the force against carbohydrate propo-

---

3.   *Protein Power* by Michael R. Eades, M.D. and Mary Dan Eades, M.D., 16, Bantam Books, page 8, footnote at bottom

nents. Eating a high carbohydrate diet is not healthy. The results of obesity and other health problems of Americans eating a high carbohydrate diet over the past century is evidence that it doesn't work. You need protein and fat. You don't need carbohydrate. That does not mean you have to completely avoid carbohydrate. You just need to minimize carbohydrate in your diet. What carbohydrates do for food is add sugar and we all like the taste of sugar. Carbohydrates are simply different units of sugar, which is the dessert of the three food groups. However, you should be eating a low carbohydrate diet to lose weight and feel healthy. And since you can live without carbohydrate, minimizing them for thirty days poses no health risks. No health problems. And you will lose weight. You will feel healthier. High protein and no more than thirty percent fat!

Protein

Protein is essential for human health as was discussed in the previous chapter. Protein can be converted to glucose, which is essential for human life and you can obtain glucose from protein through gluconeogenesis, which is the subject of the next chapter.

Protein diets are currently popular. Michael R. Eades, M.D. and Mary Dan Eades, M.D. who have written several books on nutrition write in their popular book, *Protein Power*, that eating a high protein diet is medically and nutritionally healthier than eating the traditional 60% carbohydrate diet. They point out that the 'major diseases of Western civilization—obesity, high blood pressure, heart disease, elevated blood fats, and diabetes-have a common bond…these 'diseases' aren't diseases at all, they're symptoms of a more basic single disorder, hyperinsulinemia (excess insulin) and insulin resistance…" (*Protein Power*, p.328) They recommend controlling starches and sugars and eating a high protein diet.

Robert C. Atkins, M.D., has also written a book advocating a high protein diet, which is similar to my diet books recommending 20 grams of carbohydrates a day to start and increasing your carbohydrates until you reach your 'maintenance level.' His diet is to lose weight and it works. You may read his books to confirm a diet high in protein is healthy even though other 'medical authorities' say otherwise. Here is another example of a medical doctor who legally practiced medicine advocating a high protein diet. I personally use his *Carbohydrate Gram Counter*[1] book.

This should be enough evidence to convince you that I am not alone in recommending a high protein diet, avoiding sugar, drinking lots of water and taking vitamin supplements. There are medical doctors out there and other reputable sources saying the same thing, not only for reducing obesity, but at the very least for better health. They are few, but the list is growing.

---

1. ***Dr. Atkins' New Carbohydrate Gram Counter*** by Robert C. Atkins, 1996, M.D., M. Evans and Company, Inc

If you are athletic and in good shape you probably eat a significant number of grams of carbohydrates for energy. You may experience fatigue and other problems if you switch to a high protein diet for thirty days. For some reason you have decided to change your diet so try to pick a thirty day period when you can adjust your metabolism to a high protein diet without undue physical stress that requires carbohydrate energy. After the thirty days you can evaluate what you learned from this to adjust your carbohydrate intake for energy. You should realize the benefit of reducing sugar's toxic effects on your body from this experience with a healthier body. Many of the 'energy bars' are loaded with sugar, whether it is sucrose or some other type sugar. Avoid them like the plague. Protein bars can contain more than 25 to 30 grams of carbohydrates. Avoid them too. Find protein bars with minimal or zero carbohydrates and no sugar substitutes.

Even if you are not athletic, you may experience the same thing when you change your diet from a high carbohydrate diet to a high protein diet. Some report fatigue, weakness, lethargy, or head aches. However, after a period of time your body adjusts to the high protein diet and many report better health later. Your metabolism is changing. So be patient and stick to the diet for thirty days. Don't give up just because of these aforementioned symptoms since they usually pass in time. When you change your diet your body needs to adjust and it will.

The Diet is a high protein diet for thirty days and is limited to 30 grams of carbohydrates a day. After the thirty days you can return to your high carbohydrate diet or eat all the sugar or sugar substitutes you want. What is the point of doing this for thirty days? To prove to yourself that you will lose weight or feel healthier. Sugar in your diet is not good for you. High carbohydrates must be avoided for thirty days to change your metabolism to prove this. It takes thirty days to see any significant results. When you go back to the way your were eating before changing to *The Diet* you will notice your weight or your health problems return. Eating *The Diet* works. It is only thirty days of your life. I can't convince you. You must convince yourself and the only way is to try *The Diet*.

Some complain also of constipation when changing over from a high carbohydrate diet to a high protein diet. Your metabolism is changing. You currently have an insulin dominant metabolism. To help eliminate constipation the number one solution is to drink plenty of water. Just water. Lots of water. More than you have ever drunk before. Water. Drinking large volumes of water for thirty days usually poses no health risks but I have a chapter on water you should read before you begin this diet. Also read suggestion number four in the chapter, *Ten*

Suggestions for the Thirty-Day Diet Plan, about water. Ten twelve-ounce glasses of water should be enough water if you are having problems with constipation. Second, increase the magnesium supplement to double or triple the suggested amount in the chapter *Vitamins and Supplements*. Third, increase the fish oil supplement to double or triple in the same chapter. Fourth, you need more fiber. Use Oat Bran or Flaxseed bran. You must count the carbohydrate from the bran into your daily count limit of 30 grams. A half-ounce of oat bran has 7.5 grams of carbohydrate. You can also get fiber from cabbage or other green vegetable.

Protein Synthesis and Gluconeogenesis

Many do not know what happens to the proteins you eat or the fact that you can get glucose from protein. Proteins are made up of carbon, hydrogen, and oxygen atoms combined into certain amino acids containing nitrogen. There are 22 different amino acids that your body needs, nine are essential, which means you cannot synthesize them in your body and therefore you obtain them from food. The other thirteen amino acids your body needs, the nonessential ones can be obtained from the food you eat or you can manufacture them yourself from fats, carbohydrate, and other amino acids. Basically your body uses proteins to build new cells, maintain tissues, and synthesize new proteins. Proteins from foods are broken down into their component amino acids by digestive enzymes (specialized proteins), while other enzymes inside your body cells synthesize new proteins by reassembling amino acids into specific compounds that your body needs. This process is called *protein synthesis*. About half the dietary protein you consume each day goes to make enzymes, many of which have to do with digesting food using certain vitamins and minerals for this task. New cells need protein. Nucleoproteins are chemicals in the nucleus of every living cell made up of amino acids and nucleic acids. The carbon, hydrogen, and oxygen left over after *protein synthesis* is complete is converted to glucose and used for energy. The nitrogen left over is converted to urea, most of which is excreted in urine. What *protein synthesis* does for you is wonderful since you can obtain glucose from protein that is essential for life since your cells need glucose and oxygen. You may have thought that you need glucose from carbohydrate, but the **actual amount of carbohydrate required by humans for health is zero** (see the chapter *Protein and Fat Essential for Life*). You can obtain glucose from protein through *gluconeogenesis* when amino acids are converted into glucose by the liver from non-carbohydrate food sources like protein.

Protein synthesis and gluconeogenesis effect body metabolism. This process is dependent on the liver, pancreas and other organs being in balance. What we eat can affect these organs in the way they function as a whole. If you are changing from a 60% or higher carbohydrate diet your metabolism takes time to change, possibly weeks, to release glucagon into your bloodstream and to jump-start gluconeogensis. And in time, usually about thirty days your body metabolism will adjust. You may notice some quirks in your body as you adjust from an insulin dominant metabolism to a glucagon dominant metabolism.

The high-quality proteins come from meat, fish, seafood, poultry, eggs and dairy products that are absorbed more efficiently without much waste to synthesize proteins. The proteins from plants often have limited amounts of some amino acids and our bodies do not absorb them as easily or use them as efficiently as animal proteins so their nutritional quality is considered a low-quality protein. The prime exception is the soybean, which is packed with the nine essential amino acids and is the number one source of protein for vegetarians, which is the subject of another chapter.

A high protein diet along with protein synthesis can help you control your weight and feel healthier. Gluconeogenesis manufactures the glucose you need for energy. Remember that your grandmother or your mom said that you need chicken soup when you were sick? Chicken soup is protein. It heals. That is what we need, protein.

Glucagon vs. Insulin

You may have heard of insulin but you probably have not heard of glucagon. Both hormones are made by the pancreas and regulate blood sugar. Insulin, as you probably know, enables you to digest and metabolize glucose from carbohydrate, fat or protein. Your body cells cannot burn the glucose without insulin. Impossible. Insulin is essential for human survival. If you run out of insulin you are in trouble. Doctors love to prescribe prescription insulin if your pancreas can not manufacture it anymore since insulin is essential for human survival.

Glucagon is released when blood glucose is low. Glucagon metabolizes glycogen (stored glucose) first and then the fat or protein so that body cells obtain energy. Conversion of protein into glucose was described in the chapter, *Protein Synthesis and Gluconeogenesis.*

A diet high in carbohydrate stimulates insulin production in the blood, especially when the diet includes a generous amount of sugar. This may result over time into insulin resistance in which the receptors no longer respond properly to insulin or hyperinsulinemia which means simply having too much insulin in the blood. Over time diabetes may result. While the medical authorities keep saying over and over that a sugar diet is not a factor in any of these conditions, any one with half a brain can come to the same conclusion as you just did. If 2 out of 3 diabetics suffer heart attacks or stroke it doesn't take a medical degree or a Ph.D. to understand that sugar is a factor in all these diseases. What has happened is simply eating a diet high in sugar over the years taxes the poor old pancreas who has been cranking out enormous amounts of insulin until it is simply worn out and cries 'Don't you get it? I am out of insulin!' Medical *and diet authorities* insist that eating sugar has nothing to do with diabetes, heart disease, stroke or cancer? The medical profession is ready to give you prescriptions and treatment for diabetes, heart disease or stroke.

Now the classic response is, 'What about all these people in their seventies or eighties or more who ate sugar all their life who are healthy?' My response is they are few and the majority is already either dead or is on their way out with diabetes, heart disease, stroke, cancer or some other disease. If you take a revolver with one bullet in the chamber of six slots, spin it and then click it to your head you have a one in six possibility that the gun will go off and kill or hurt you. Now take that gun and hand it to the next fellow and do this for millions of people over seventy or eighty years. Sure, there will be a few still alive in their seventy and eighties. But how many were shot? Would you accept that gun and pull the trigger to your head? Many do when they eat sugar in such huge quantities. When you eat sugar in your diet along with a high carbohydrate diet you are wearing your pancreas out trying to make insulin. Remember that insulin is essential for human life. You need it. You only have so much to make and then, poof, no more. The *Sugar Age* began at the beginning of the eighteenth century. When humans ate food before the advent of the *Sugar Age* the pancreas could handle the carbohydrate the average human ate. Before the *Sugar Age* diabetes was rare. With the advent of the *Sugar Age* diabetes, heart disease, stroke, and cancer have risen in greater percentages since 1700. Sugar is a factor in these diseases without a doubt.

The pancreas releases glucagon when your blood glucose is low. After burning up all the glycogen, glucagon starts working on fat and protein breaking it down to glucose to burn in your cells. You want to have a glucagon dominate metabolism. No doubt before the *Sugar Age* mankind's metabolism was glucagon dominate. Since the *Sugar Age* began mankind has steadily changed over from bodies that were glucagon dominant to an insulin dominant metabolism. You need to save every drop of insulin you have left. Think of this formula:

L = your life span
X = amount of insulin your pancreas can make
D = your diet

L = X/D

God only knows what your pancreas can make over a lifetime of eating all the sugar you consume along with a high carbohydrate diet. You will eventually know yourself when the doctor says you have diabetes. You think you can be one of the few who make it into the eighties eating and drinking sugar the whole way with your little 'ole pancreas pumping its little heart out squeezing the last bit of insulin it has to produce for your sugar sweet life? Go for it. Pull the trigger and you are wiping out your pancreas. But what if you are not one of the few who make it into your seventies or eighties with a healthy pancreas?

And quality of life is not in the above formula until you develop diabetes, heart disease, cancer, stroke or something else. You want to try factoring that in? Treatment for these diseases is not fun and your quality of life isn't what it used to be if you get any of these diseases.

If sugar is a factor in these diseases, no doubt there is a long list of other diseases in which sugar is a factor. And you don't think diabetes is serious. It is dead serious. Remember that two our three diabetics die of heart disease or stroke. Many die of cancer. On the death certificates of these diabetics who die of heart disease, stroke or cancer do you think the cause of death is diabetes? No the certificate lists heart disease, stroke or cancer and the statistics show these as the leading cause of death. The current number of people with diabetes worldwide is 170 million in 2003. Will you be the next one added to this statistic?

When you eat a low carbohydrate diet you will need insulin to metabolize the glucose. You want it available. You shouldn't want prescription insulin that comes from a prescription. You want the real insulin made by your own pancreas. One possibility you may assure you have insulin is to have a glucagon dominant blood metabolism. Right now you probably have an insulin dominant metabolism. To change your metabolism will cost you. What will it cost? Your suffering this change with a thirty-day diet suggested in this book. The cost is well worth it. Your weight will drop and you will feel healthier. In thirty days you will have a glucagon dominate metabolism and notice the big difference in your weight loss and health if you follow the 30-day diet plan in this book. You are the *diet authority* and can choose whether you want a glucagon dominant metabolism or let your insulin dominance remain the same and see if you make it into your seventies or eighties healthy. I think the odds are against those with an insulin dominant metabolism. Seriously consider insulin vs. glucagon. Glucagon should win. You are the only one who can help glucagon win.

Fat vs. Sugar

Something needs to be said about concerns over sugar vs. fat. For years the medical profession and nutritionists have warned that fat is bad for your health with very little concern about sugar. You have to decide if you can stop worrying about fat for thirty days to see if *The Diet* controls your weight and you feel healthier. After the thirty days, you can avoid all the fat you want especially which type of fat. Just remember that all health authorities say that you may have up to 30 percent of your total calories from fat, which amounts to 66.7 grams of fat in a 2000-calorie diet! (See the chapter *Protein and Fat—Essential for Life*) If you take my suggestion to read *Protein Power* you will discover that the 'fat is bad' myth is just that, a myth. *The Diet* will actually lower your 'bad' cholesterol and raise your 'good' cholesterol levels. What is bad is eating sugar, highly refined processed food, or a diet high in carbohydrates. Over the years this taxes your body's immune system or upsets your metabolism to a point of being unable to cope with diseases like diabetes or other vascular disorders. Eating sugar in your diet is more of a concern than eating fat. Mankind has consumed sugar and refined carbohydrates in processed food in such huge quantities only for the last couple of hundred years or so when sugarcane from the West Indies began to be shipped to the rest of the world. Before this, mankind had a diet that mainly consisted of meat, fish, fowl, dairy, eggs, grains, vegetables, fruits and very little honey or maple syrup. Sweets were just not available in the amount consumed today. Sucrose in the form of a white crystal was not known for thousands of years! But for the last couple of hundred years or so, sugar consumption has grown at an astronomical rate. NEVER has mankind eaten the amount of sugar that the world consumes now. The typical American eats 149 pounds of sugar a year! That is right, ONE HUNDRED FORTY NINE pounds! And the *diet authorities* keep saying that heart disease and diabetes, which are vascular disorders, have little to do with sugar, and fat is the culprit? These authorities point to FAT as the problem and continue to say that SUGAR is hardly a worry. Heart disease is still the number one killer for Americans and diabetes is the tenth leading cause of death, even though the medical authorities bless low fat diets. For millenniums mankind has not had to use the pancreas to produce the amount of insulin required to eat the amount of sugar the average American eats. When sugar was not eaten in such huge quantity mankind gave little concern about eating fat. It is only in the twentieth century that the medical authorities became concerned over fat, with barely a concern over the sugar consumption in such huge amounts. History may show someday that the large amount of sugar consumption during this period was a factor in many of the diseases resulting from an insulin dominant metabolism. So you have to decide, fat verses sugar for thirty days. Just enjoy the protein and whatever fat comes along with it. It's only thirty days. You can go back to worrying about fat after the thirty days. What you should worry about is sugar in your diet, not fat. And what if *The Diet* really controls your weight and you feel healthier? The only way to know is try it for thirty days. And I urge you again to please read *Protein Power* and *Sugar Busters!* Protein is actually good for you and will help control your weight and you will feel healthier. This is what *The Diet* is all about. When using oil, I recommend Extra Virgin Olive Oil, all natural cold pressed. Thirty days eating a high protein diet along with whatever fat comes with it is not a health risk.

Vitamins and Supplements

Daily Vitamin Supplements Suggested

Acidophilus (40,000,000 CFU three times a day or more)
Vitamin A—25,000 IU
High Potency B Complex—1 tab/capsule
Flush Free Niacin [B-3] (Inositol Hexanicotinate)—100 mg
Pantothenic Acid [B-5]—100mg
B-6—50 mg
B-12—250 mcg.
Beta Carotene—25,000 IU
Calcium-at least 1000 mg
Zinc—15 mg
Vitamin C [at least 500—suggest 1000 to 3000 mg] (*Ester-C*™ recommended)
Vitamin D—400 I.U.
Vitamin E—400 I.U.
Evening Primrose—1000 mg.
Fish Oil—1000 mg
Grape Seed Extract—50 mg
Glucosamine Complex—1.5 g
L-Lysine—1000 mg
Mangesium—399 mg
MSM (Methylsulfonylmethane)—1000 mg
Multivitamin—1 tab
Pantothenic Acid—500 mg
Potassium—1100 mg
Selenium—200 mcg

These are the minimum suggested

More vitamins are your choice. By taking vitamins, it will help curb your appetite
for sweets. And in a few weeks you will notice the difference they can make in

your life. My personal theory is that we need the extra vitamin supplements since the processed food in our diet lacks nutrients and we need the boost since an insulin dominant metabolism has been leaching our vitamins and minerals. If you decide to take these suggestions always consume vitamins and supplements at breakfast with your food. If you take some vitamins at night, you may not sleep well, so try to take them at breakfast or lunch, always with food. There is some controversy with vitamins, and I don't want to debate on this subject. If you have an issue with any of the above suggestions, remember that the above vitamins/minerals are just a suggestion. I buy most of my vitamins at Wal-Mart or Costco. Some complain that vitamins are costly but give no thought to the cost of junk food, candy or milk shakes. If you cut out the sugar and junk food for thirty days the money you save should more than compensate the investment of vitamin and mineral supplements I suggest. You will not believe how the vitamins and minerals suggested would improve your health and give you the boost you need for energy unless you try it. Whatever the cost, it is only for thirty days and after that you can decide yourself if the money you spent on vitamins and minerals was worth it. To give you an idea of the cost of this my wife and I spend about $75 a month for two people on vitamins and supplements in 2003! How much do you spend for dinner out at a nice restaurant? So you can't sacrifice one restaurant meal during this month you are trying *The Diet*? If money is still the issue then do the best you can with vitamins. The amount of vitamins I suggest taking doesn't have to be set in stone. You can alter the suggestions according to what brand you buy and figure it out for your situation.

I also suggest you take the following vitamins just before bed with a glass of water:
Acidophilus (40,000,000 CFU)
L-Lysine—500 mg
Calcium—1000 mg
Magnesium—399 mg
Zinc—15 mg
Potassium—1100 mg
Vitamin C—1000 mg. (*Ester-C*™ recommended)

Water

Water is essential for human survival. We get water from the food and drink we consume. What is the minimum amount of water essential for good health? There is considerable variation here due to individual sweating rates, body size and weight, heat and humidity, and running speed, and other factors[1]. However it is generally believed that for the average adult two liters of water a day is recommended[2]. Your individual condition determines how much water you may need to lose weight and feel healthier. But you may not be getting enough water with your current diet and I recommend more water than you may be currently drinking.

During the thirty-days of *The Diet* I suggest drinking at least eight glasses of twelve-ounces of water and if possible drinking ten glasses. Most health authorities recommend drinking eight glasses of eight ounces of water per day. I prefer twelve ounces because you can visualize a twelve-ounce container. An eight-ounce container is not easily visualized since they are rare. I think you need more water for health or to lose weight.

Some may be concerned about drinking this much water, which is a valid concern. You can not be drinking too much water unless you have a disease state like kidney, heart disease, or some other condition. I have explained in my legal disclaimer that you should not begin this diet without consulting your physician. Excess water normally will be passed out of the body by urinating, sweating, defecating, and exhaling thereby preventing fluid retention. A condition known as

---

1. "The primary determinant of maintenance water requirement appears to be metabolic (Holliday and Segar, 1957), but the actual estimation of water requirement is highly variable and quite complex. Because the water requirement is the amount necessary to balance the insensible losses (which can vary markedly) and maintain a tolerable solute load for the kidneys (which may vary with dietary composition and other factors), it is impossible to set a general water requirement." Source > http://books.nap.edu/books/0309046335/html/249.html#pagetop
2. http://www.i-medreview.com/articles_html/nutritionwellness/essnutrients.html

hyponatremia[3]—sometimes called water intoxication—is caused when levels of sodium in the blood drop to dangerously low levels. However, this condition is rare and usually found in extreme cases, such as long distance runners who drink copious amounts of water without replenishing sodium or electrolytes resulting in the body's salt and water levels getting dangerously out of balance. It leads to swelling of the brain and leakage of fluid into the lungs. Remember that this condition is rare and extreme.

The range I suggest is between 96 ounces of water per day to a maximum of 120 ounces. This amounts to between two and a half liters to a little over three liters of water per day. For thirty days this usually will pose no health problems. If you have some health condition causing you water retention or some other health concern discuss your water intake and diet with your health care practitioner. Our kidneys are equipped to efficiently process fifteen liters of water a day. That's equivalent to drinking about sixty glasses of water! I am not recommending sixty glasses of water. Excess water we take in that is not needed is usually passed out as urine within a few hours if everything is working satisfactorily.

By most current dietetic standards, the guideline is that most healthy adults normally require approximately three quarts of fluid each day. Half of the liquid comes from food and the other half from what you drink. Drinking 8 to 12 glasses a day of eight-ounce containers should be sufficient for keeping your system in good working order. But I recommend more since I think you need to flush your system to lose weight and feel healthier when changing over from an insulin dominant metabolism to a glucagon dominant one.

In the thirty-day plan I have suggested when to drink a glass of 12 ounces of water in ten suggested times a day for each day of the diet. Not juice, soft drinks, just water! If you can't drink that much water, remember this is just a suggestion and you are the *diet authority* and can drink whatever amount you want or drink the amount recommended by your health practitioner. You may find that drinking the amount of water I suggest will help you lose weight and feel healthier.

---

3.   "Toxicity results from the ingestion of water at a rate beyond the capacity of the kidneys to excrete the extra load, resulting in hyposmolarity. Such a condition is rarely observed in a normal healthy adult. The manifestations usually include a gradual mental dulling, confusion, coma, convulsion, and even death." Source > http://books.nap.edu/books/0309046335/html/250.html#pagetop

Puzzling Pyramids

Before the USDA came out with its famous Food Guide Pyramid in 1992, the typical American ate 40% Fat, 15% Protein, and 45% Carbohydrate[1]. If you like, go to this url and check out the Food Guide and try to figure out the percentages that the government recommended to the public in 1992 >

http://www.pueblo.gsa.gov/cic_text/food/food-pyramid/main.htm

If you can figure it out you are one smart cookie. The only percentage mentioned is the famous 30% fat figure. That is why I call it a puzzling pyramid. Who can understand it? Servings? What does that mean? My wife may serve her plate and I would still be hungry if I ate her servings. What percentage of protein should I eat? What percentage of carbohydrate should I eat? Another puzzle is how the USDA Pyramid breaks food up. It breaks all food into six categories:

Fats, Oils and Sweets-Use Sparingly
Milk, Yogurt, Cheese Group—2 to 3 Servings
Meat, Poultry, Fish, Dry beans, Eggs & Nuts Group—2 to 3 Servings
Vegetable Group—3 to 5 Servings
Fruit Group—2 to 4 Servings
Grain Group—5–11 Servings

Ok, where is a McDonald's hamburger in this pyramid? What about a pepperoni pizza? Are you puzzled? The brochure that the government provides to explain this pyramid is more puzzling. If you note at the top of the pyramid that fat is to be used sparingly yet the brochure says that your total fat can be up to 30%. Is that confusing to you? That makes this pyramid contradictory if the tiny top of the pyramid allows 30% of your total caloric intake. I can make it more puzzling but you can at least see why most Americans ignore this Pyramid. The bottom

---

1. *Scientific American*, January 2003, *Rebuilding the Food Pyramid*, Walter C. Willett and Meir J. Stampfer

line is that the USDA Food Guide Pyramid is approximately 60% Carbohydrate, 25% Fat, and 15% Protein.

As Newsweek magazine pointed out, Americans ignore this pyramid and eat what they want and have chosen to eat more sweets and meat. The typical American Diet works out to approximately 75% Carbohydrate, 15% Protein, and 10% Fat. What the USDA Food Guide Pyramid accomplished was to change the American way of eating before 1992 from eating 40% fat to 10% and instead of eating more protein everyone ate more carbohydrates.

The USDA is planning on revising the Food Guide Pyramid and it is reported to be released sometime in 2004[2]. There are other pyramids like the NEW FOOD GUIDE PYRAMID mentioned in the preceding footnote, the Mediterranean Food Pyramid, the Asian Food Pyramid and probably others you may have heard of. I still find them all puzzling. What I find easier to understand is not pyramids but percentages. You can imagine the three food groups in your mind right now, can't you? So let's discuss percentages.

Just about all the health authorities say you can eat up to 30% Fat. So starting with this as a base lets figure out in our minds what should be the percentages of proteins and fats. An easy way to do this is simply divide the three groups into thirds and each group would be 33 per cent. Based on the current nutritional research splitting it three ways equally is better than the typical American diet which has raised obesity.

The authorities point out that the MINIMUM requirement of protein to survive is somewhere between 50 to 100 grams. You think you just want to eat the minimum, or should we eat more for better health? Duh? We need protein. You need protein to heal, build, and grow. We don't need carbohydrates. Carbohydrates are like dessert that make life enjoyable. We need to maximize our protein intake, not maximize our carbohydrate. A good goal is to eat at least 50% protein, 20% for carbohydrates. Doesn't that make sense?

The thirty-day diet in this book (based on a 2000 calorie a day diet) is:

64% PROTEIN—30% FAT—6% CARBOHYDRATE

---

2.   *Scientific American*, January 2003, *Rebuilding the Food Pyramid*, Walter C. Willett and Meir J. Stampfer

The Diet is extreme for thirty days to change your insulin dominant metabolism over to a glucagon dominant one. AFTER the thirty days you can then experiment all you want with the percentages of the three basic food groups. The thirty-day diet is to prove you can lose weight and feel healthier with a high protein diet.

The debate over these percentages will go on and on. You are the *diet authority* and you can decide your own percentages. The other debate is what protein, fat and carbohydrate to eat. Fix in mind that protein should be at the top of the percentage, not carbohydrate. That is what should be in your mind and the puzzling pyramids can stay in Egypt where they ought to be.

Sugar Suffice Is Not Nice

Sugar and spice and everything nice. Sugar suffice is not nice.

The above two statements cannot be both true. You have been conditioned by mom and the processed food industry that sugar is nice. Sugar is not nice. Sugar is toxic.

Sugar Busters! by H. Leighton Steward, Morrison C. Bethea, M.D., Samuel S. Andrews, M.D., and Luis A Balart, M.D. states on page 17 that "**SUGAR IS TOXIC!**" Three of the authors are medical doctors and recommend a low-sugar diet, avoiding carbohydrates with a high glycemic index. Do you get it? Medical doctors are saying that sugar is toxic. How can they write a book stating that sugar is toxic and still be licensed physicians? That is because it is true, sugar is toxic and is cumulative over time.

William Dufty summarizes the toxic effect of sugar in his book, *Sugar Blues*, when he kicked the habit. Dufty threw all the sugar in his kitchen out and just ate grains and vegetables. He wrote,

> In about forty-eight hours, I was in total agony, overcome with nausea, with a crashing migraine. If pain was a message, this was a long one, very involved, intense but in code. It took hours to break the code. I knew enough about junkies to recognize reluctantly my kinship with them. I was kicking cold turkey, the thing they talked about with such terror. After all, heroin is nothing but a chemical. They take the juice of the poppy and they refine it into opium and then they refine it to morphine and finally to heroin. Sugar is nothing but a chemical. They take the juice of the cane or the beet and they refine it to molasses and then they refine it to brown sugar and finally to strange white crystals. It's no wonder dope pushers dilute pure heroin with milk sugar—lactose—in order to make their glassine packages a treat to the eye. I was kicking all kinds of chemicals cold turkey—sugar, aspirin, cocaine, caffeine, chlorine, fluorine, sodium, monosodium glutamate, and all those other multisyllabic horrors listed in fine print on the tins and boxes I had just thrown in the trash. I had it very rough for about twenty-four hours, but the morning after was a

revelation. I went to sleep with exhaustion, sweating and tremors. I woke up feeling reborn."[1]

You may or may not experience such withdrawals depending on how much you are addicted to sugar. Dufty ate a high carbohydrate diet when he went off sugar which was at the very least better than eating a diet full of sugar. Eating a high carbohydrate diet helps reduce the addictive withdrawal symptoms of getting off sugar. Carbohydrates are units of different type sugar. If you eat the 'typical American diet' that includes 149 pounds of sugar a year, addiction to sugar is no doubt the reason many cannot stop eating sugar.

Nicholas V. Perricone, M.D., has books on how to have healthy skin and offers a number of skin care products. He also advocates a diet eating foods low in the glycemic index, avoiding refined and packaged sugar, drinking plenty of water, taking his suggested supplements, and eating fish protein. His two more popular books are *The Wrinkle Cure* and *The Perricone Prescription*. He is a licensed dermatologist. In one of his newsletters, *Dr. Perricone Skin Science Update Newsletter*, Dr. Perricone quotes some research done by the American Diabetes Association as follows,

> "…The results of several related studies presented at the June, 2002 meeting of the American Diabetes Association confirm my own finding that high-glycemic carbohydrates—sugars and starchy foods such as pasta, potatoes, and bread—cause an inflammatory response that accelerates aging and contributes to a variety of diseases (heart disease, some types of cancer, arthritis, Alzheimer's, etc.). In addition, one of the studies showed that the antioxidant vitamins E and C block this inflammatory response. The results of the new studies support the conclusions of a prior study showing that dietary sugars increase blood levels of free radicals and pro-inflammatory enzymes to a greater degree than foods that are high in fat or protein…"

In his book, *The Wrinkle Cure*, (Warner Books) Dr. Perricone states on page 10,

> "When you consume carbohydrates, your blood sugar begins to rise and insulin is secreted by your pancreas to keep that sugar under control. The problem is that the release of insulin pushes your cellular metabolism into a mode in which it produces inflammatory chemicals…This whole process is very nicely described by Barry Sears, M.D., in his book *Enter the Zone* (HarperCollins, 15). Dr. Sears explains that insulin, in high levels, tends to create chemicals in

---

1.   *Sugar Blues*, William Dufty, 1975, Warner Books, Inc, p. 22–3

the body that encourage inflammation. The result is not only prematurely aged skin, but also degenerative diseases such as heart disease, cancer, Alzheimer's and many other illnesses.

The best way to be sure that your insulin levels are under control is to eat foods that are low on the glycemic index..."

Actually the quote above refers to Barry Sears as a medical doctor, but Barry Sears is actually a Ph.D., not a medical doctor. Dr. Perricone recognizes sugar's toxic effects. He discusses a process known as glycation when sugar attaches to proteins and become cross-linked resulting in sagging and inflexible skin (page 7). He states on page 72 of his book that the 'real answer is to eat less sugar,' and recommends his 'anti-inflammatory diet.' He also discusses on page 105 how sugar interacts with collagen in a process known as glycosylation and says, "you're much better off…dropping the added sugar from your diet."

William Dufty wrote on page 175 of his book,

> "It is mind boggling today to read through medical histories and other tomes and find again and again that the basic cause of diabetes mellitus is still unknown, that it is chronic and incurable, or that it is due to the failure of the pancreas to secrete an adequate amount of insulin. It's still Greek to the best of them."[2]

In 2003 on the American Diabetes Association's website, when you click on Basic Diabetes Information, you may read this statement:

> "The cause of diabetes continues to be a mystery, although both genetics and environmental factors such as obesity and lack of exercise appear to play roles."

This gives you an idea of how the mainstream health authorities appear to be clueless to diet's connection with disease. But you do see the connection don't you? The above quote says obesity plays a factor in diabetes. Duh, could diet be a factor in diabetes?

Remember that 2 out of 3 people with diabetes die from heart disease and stroke? Does diet play a factor in heart disease and stroke? Now it was possible to go to

---

2.   *Sugar Blues*, William Dufty, 1975, Warner Books, Inc, p. 77–8

the ADA's site on diabetes in 2003 and look for the Frequently Asked Questions and read what the second most frequently asked question is. Guess? Here it is:

"Can I eat foods with sugar in them?"

The answer according to the American Diabetes Association:

"For almost every person with diabetes, the answer is yes! Eating a piece of cake made with sugar will raise your blood glucose level. So will eating corn on the cob, a tomato sandwich, or lima beans. The truth is that sugar has gotten a bad reputation. People with diabetes can and do eat sugar. In your body, it becomes glucose, but so do the other foods mentioned above. With sugary foods, the rule is moderation. Eat too much, and 1) you'll send your blood glucose level up higher than you expected; 2) you'll fill up but without the nutrients that come with vegetables and grains; and 3) you'll gain weight. So, don't pass up a slice of birthday cake. Instead, at the next meal, eat a little less bread or potato and be sure to take a brisk walk to burn some calories."
source > http://www.diabetes.org/nutrition/faqs.asp#SugarFoods

Medical authorities agree that persons with diabetes are at a higher risk for heart disease. Yet connecting sugar consumption over the years to either disease is over-looked, minimized or lacking by these medical authorities. If you look at a graph published in the book *Sugar Busters!*, it shows how the consumption of sugar has climbed dramatically only in the last couple of centuries. Now compare this with a graph on the dramatic climb of diabetes during this same period, it doesn't take a clinical study to see the connection. The damage of high sugar consumption to a person's body not only effects diseases like diabetes and heart disease but possibly is a major factors in many other diseases. Remember 170 million people on this planet have diabetes and the number continues to rise!

While the USDA's Food Pyramid 'balanced food group' diet limits sugar, the pyramid still blesses sugar consumption in small amounts at the top of the pyramid.

Obesity is now the culprit used by medical authorities as being the factor for several major diseases. Does diet play a factor in obesity? Sugar causes obesity. Reducing sugar in your diet will reduce obesity. Eliminating sugar from your diet promotes health and well being.

Weight loss will result when you reduce sugar in your diet. How does this happen? Your body breaks down all food into glucose so that the cells can use the energy and live. Any excess glucose is converted to glycogen ("animal starch") and stored in your liver, muscles and blood to be used if needed. This is a wonderful storehouse of packed energy that can easily be converted back to glucose when needed. There is one problem. The body can only store about 14 ounces of glycogen or about 400 grams[3]. A gram of glucose has four calories. The entire amount of stored glycogen is approximately 1600 to 1800 calories. Since there is limited glycogen storage, if your diet includes a generous amount of sugars and carbohydrates and your glycogen storehouse is full, the excess sugars and carbohydrates will be converted to **FAT** and the body gains weight. *The Diet* stops this excess conversion of sugars and carbohydrates into fat, thus resulting in weight loss over time. This is just one of the reasons why sugar should be avoided in your diet not to mention you will feel healthier!

Refined sugar [sucrose] in crystallized form is artificial usually made from either sugar beets or sugarcane. Some may claim that sugar is natural, but would you call the crystallized powder heroin derived from morphine 'natural,' because it is made from the opium of a poppy? Refined table sugar doesn't occur naturally, it is an artificially manufactured process. I toured a sugar plantation and factory in Kauai, Hawaii this year and saw the process how sugar cane is made into raw sugar. Lime is used. What is done to raw sugar to make this product into a pure white crystal? There is no way you can call this natural. It is a manufactured processed artificial sugar reducing the sugar cane plant into an addictive pure white crystal not unlike how the poppy flower is used to make opium into morphine and heroine. This process is a manufacturing artificial process not found in nature. You simply do not find these white crystals called sugar or heroine in nature.

You may have no idea how the processed food industry has adulterated most of the food and drink you are consuming with sucrose or some other type sugar. Remember that the typical American eats 149 pounds of it a year! And the typical American diet is being promoted all over the world to eat and as a result sugar is being consumed in greater quantities each year worldwide—so is diabetes, heart disease, and cancer. And if it wasn't for people like Ralph Nador you wouldn't see the sugar content on the label of the food and drink you buy in the U.S.A.

---

3.   Nutrition For Dummies ®, 1997, Carol Ann Rinzler, IDG Books Worldwide, Inc., p. 81

For example, even the sucrose contained in one teaspoon of catsup on French Fries not to mention the starch (which is another form of sugar) in the French Fries is loaded with carbohydrate. One teaspoon of Catsup has 3.8 grams of carbohydrates! Ten French Fries has 18 grams of carbohydrates, mostly starch. That is just one example of carbohydrate in your diet. What all this sugar and a diet high in carbohydrate have done to your health is manifesting as obesity and other diseases.

Just about any dentist will tell you sugar is the cause of cavities in your teeth. If you stop eating sugar, it may not help the cavity already developed in your tooth, but will help control or prevent other cavities from forming. Does that mean you will not ever get a cavity again if you never eat sugar again? Well, no, you might get one, but your chances are drastically reduced to practically zero. Most dentists will tell you that as long as you brush your teeth and avoid sugar you will reduce your cavity possibilities to near zero. Have you noticed how many people are losing their teeth and how much sugar they consume? Dentists know the connection sugar has with rotten teeth. They are only glad to replace your teeth with artificial ones. Do you really think that cavities are the only thing 'rotten' in your body from all the sugar you have been eating over your lifetime?

You may ask, 'if sugar is so bad for your health, why do the health or *diet authorities* minimize the toxic effects of sugar?' The *Sugar Buster!* authors put it this way on page 36–37 of their book,

> "…Pro-sugar lobbying by sugar growers, cola manufactures and the packaged-food industry has been very effective in influencing our government. What politician wants to tell his constituents they should no longer eat sugar?"

Why do health 'authorities' continue to bless sugar? Another reason may be the quote below:

> "The American Dietetic Association, which trains registered dieticians to direct preparation of hospital and institutional food, has been soundly criticized for its association with the Sugar Association and companies like Coca Cola and M&M Mars. Such groups supply about 15% of the ADA's annual budget…"[4]

---

4. *Nourishing Traditions*, Sally Fallon with Mary G. Enig, Ph.D, New Trends Publishing, 1999, P. 571

Sugar is big business. It permeates the food industry. If you think the tobacco industry is powerful, the sugar industry is just as entrenched powerfully in the world's economy if not more so. Even if it reached the point of a warning label of sugar's toxic effects like the tobacco industry has been forced to use on its product, people will continue to eat sugar just as those who smoke ignore the warning label. Only people who care about their health will be motivated enough to remove sugar from their diet.

There is so much information on the web or in your public library showing the harmful effects of sugar. Just go to any major search engine and type in 'sugar' in the search box and you will be amazed at the results. Or spend a few hours at your local library. I have chosen some books and these two urls as examples:

Dangers of Sugar
78 Ways Sugar Can Ruin Your Health
http://www.mercola.com/article/sugar/

Refined sugar—the sweetest poison of all
http://www.askwaltstollmd.com/archives/sugar/5283.html
http://www.bcn.net/~stoll/sugarimm.html

Sugar Busters! by H. Leighton Steward, Dr. Morrison C. Bethea, Dr. Samued Dr. Luis A Balart, 15, *Sugar Busters!*, LLC, Figure 2, page 3 shows a graph that in 1996 the total refined sugar consumption per person per year in the USA was 149 pounds—How much did you consume over your life that has damaged your health and caused you to gain weight? On page 17 of the same publication you need to be convinced what the authors state, that "**SUGAR IS TOXIC!**" *Consumption of sugar may be hazardous to your health* may not be on food labels any time soon but more medical authorities are making such statements like these courageous doctors have done in their book.

There are a number of articles and books you may read on this subject which are listed below or can be found on the web:

Pure, White and Deadly, John Yudkin, Viking, 186, Penguin, 188, Davis-Poynter Ltd; ASIN: 070670006

Sweet and Dangerous: The New Facts About the Sugar You Eat As a Cause of Heart Disease, Diabetes, and Other Killers. by John Yudkin

Metabolic Effects of Utilizable Dietary Carbohydrates by Sheldon Reiser (Editor) (Hardcover—August 1982)

The Saccharine Disease: Conditions Caused by the taking of Refined Carbohydrates, such as sugar and white flour by T. L. Cleave

Dismantling a Myth: The Role of Fat and Carbohydrates in Our Diet by Wolfgang Lutz

Refined Carbohydrate Foods and Disease: Some Implications of Dietary Fiber by D. Burkitt

Are you beginning to understand that *sugar suffice is not nice*!

Sugars to Avoid

This chapter should be used to refer when you are using the thirty-day diet plan for vegetarians or omnivores. The Nutrition Facts Label appearing on all USA products sold in America can be used to find the total amount of carbohydrates in a product. If you are in another country hopefully there is something on the product that lists something. There is also a list of ingredients usually on every USA product that may list sugars used. Both of these can be used to figure out if sugar is in a product, first the **Nutrition Facts Label** and second, the LIST OF INGREDIENTS. Keep in mind the food process industry has figured out ways to hide the sugar in a product. You have to be smart to figure whether a product has sugar in it to avoid the product for thirty days. Of course, you as the *diet authority* can eat as much sugar as you want, but I am suggesting you avoid this entire list of sugars for thirty days to see if you lose weight or feel healthier. At the end of the thirty days you may decide to avoid sugar for life!

I think I have compiled one of the longest list of sugars used by the processed food industry which keeps finding new ways to add sugar to your life. This list is by no means complete because as soon as I publish this current list I find new ones. What I suggest is that you at least read the list. This will give you an idea of how invasive sugar has become in the processed food industry in all its various forms. After all, carbohydrate is simply different units of sugar so it is only a matter of breaking some food down into a simple sugar to be added to a product so it tastes sweeter and you buy it. If you find one not on this list, please join The Diet Users Support Group and post it so I can add it to a future revision of this book. I also keep a current list of the Sugars to Avoid in a file on the yahoo group site for you to read.

SUGAR TO AVOID

(For thirty days avoid the following sugars which may appear on any list of ingredients)

Agave Nectar
Arabinose
Apricot nectar
Barley malt
Beet Sugar
Blackstrap Molasses
Brown Sugar
Cane Juice
Cane Sugar
Corn Sweetner
Corn Syrup
Corn solids
Dark brown sugar molasses
Date Sugar
Dextrose (an optical isomer of glucose which is dextrorotatory)
Evaporated cane juice
Fruit Juice Concentrate (any type fruit—apple, pear, grape, etc.)
Fructooligosaccharides
Fructose ($CH_2OH(CHOH)_3COCH_2OH$)
Galactose; ($C_6H_{12}O_6$)
Glucose ($C_6H_{12}O_6$)
Glycogen
High Fructose Corn Syrup (HFCS)
Honey
Invert Sugar (50:50 fructose-glucose)
Lactose ($C_{12}H_{22}O_{11}$)
Levulose
Maltose
Maltodextrin
Mannose
Maple Syrup
Molasses
Monosaccharides

Muscovado (Natural light brown muscovado sugar)
Organic sugar
Organic powdered sugar
Papaya Nectar
Peach Nectar
Polycose
Polydextrose
Polysaccarides
Powdered sugar
Raffinose
Rapadura
Raw Sugar
Rice syrup
Sorghum
Starch
Stachyose
sucanat
Sucrose (C12H22O11)
Sugar Cane Juice
Sugar Cane natural organic Sucanat
Sugar crystals
Syrup (any type no matter what)
Turbinado Sugar
Turbino
Unsulfured Molasses
Xylose

All Sugar Substitutes are to be avoided for thirty days such as:

Acesulfame-K
Acesulfame Potassium
Alitame
Aspartame
Cyclamates
Equal
Lo Han
Luo Han Guo Fruit extract
Neotame
Nutrisweet

Saccharin
Splenda
Stevia
Stevia plus fiber
Sucralose
Sweet and Slender

Sugar Alcohols to avoid:

Hydrogenated Starch Hydrolysates (HSH)
Isomalt
Lactitol
Maltitol
Mannitol
Sorbitol
Xylitol

For more information on sugar substitutes go to this url >

http://www.cfsan.fda.gov/~dms/fdsugar.html

http://www.aspartemekills.com

The sugar alcohols-xylitol, mannitol, and sorbitol have some calories or carbohydrate that slightly increase blood glucose level. Avoid anything that says 'syrup' whether corn syrup or 'any' syrup! Some sugar substitutes may have carbohydrate so look at the Nutrition Facts Label and note any carbohydrate or sugar grams. Watch out for maltitol and corn syrup solids. **NO SUGAR SUBSTITUES** even if it has ZERO sugars or carbohydrate for thirty days, **NONE**. It doesn't matter whatever name it is called, whether calorie-free sweeteners like Nutrisweet, Splenda, Equal, aspartame, saccharin, and acesulfame-K**, NO SUGAR SUBSTITUTES**—AFTER the thirty days you can experiment with sugar substitutes all you want. You will figure out if your health suffers by this simple thirty-day experiment of avoiding sugar substitutes. You will know if you can use them or not when you try them again, no matter what the health authorities say about the safety of these sugar substitutes. Remember that you are the *diet authority*, not anyone else.

Some have found that certain sugar substitutes trigger allergic reactions or cause health problems. The real reason for no sugar substitutes for thirty days is so you can taste sugar in your food and drink, to be able to detect it! If you are sprinkling or adding sugar substitutes to your food or drink during the 30 Day Diet Plan, there is no way for you to be able to taste if sugar is somehow present in any of the food or drink you consume. Consequently you will then be more sensitive to the taste of sugar in your food or drink to avoid it for the 30 Days.

AFTER the thirty days, you may experiment all you want. First, prove to yourself that *The Diet* does CONTROL your weight and helps you feel healthier! You will be surprised at how sensitive you become in detecting sugar in your food and drink and how it creeps into processed food and drink. Most sugar substitutes are processed from sugar and are just as unhealthy for you as sugar, if not more so. What do you think the long-term health risks are from sugar substitutes? You will find out if you use them.

So if you have to use a sugar substitute **AFTER the 30-day Diet plan**, I recommend **Stevia**, a natural leaf that is 300 times sweeter than sugar with zero carbohydrate grams found in health stores. Who knows what the long-term use of **Stevia** may do to you but you may be able to use it instead of sugar or sugar substitutes and be healthier? So Stevia is my recommendation and you will just have to live with the health consequences. Some have claimed that Stevia poses no health risks. One thing I have found with Stevia is less is more. The more Stevia the worse it tastes. The less Stevia the better it tastes. You can find out more information on Stevia by typing in stevia into any search engine and boom you get more information that you can handle. The one fact about Stevia that is interesting is that *Coca-Cola®* used stevia in *Diet Coke®* in Japan for a period of time and was popular. Due to a corporate decision it was dropped and another sugar substitute was used which effected the production of *Diet Coke®* worldwide. I think I would try *Diet Coke®* if it had Stevia in it instead of whatever is in it now! But you can see from this how economic corporate decisions effect your choice of food and drink. But you have a choice whether to buy the product or avoid it.

Sweet Leaf Stevia Plus Fiber contains a packet that has less than 1 gram of carbohydrate per serving. More info at >

http://www.steviaplus.com

An alternative is Sweet and Slender Natural sweetener made from fructose and Luo Han Guo fruit extract that contains less than one gram of carbohydrate per packet. Both of these products can be found at the following urls >

http://www.sweetandslender.com
http://www.wisdomherbs.com

Another product made by Renew Life is SweetLife made from fructose, Lo Han and fructooligosaccharides which has one gram of carbohydrates per gram serving.

My recommendation is avoid all other sugar substitutes and sugar for the rest of your life but since you are the *diet authority*, you choose. It may be possible that some of the sugar substitutes mentioned above might not pose any health problems but I don't recommend eating 149 pounds of the product in a year. Moderation in sugar substitutes is obvious.

Prove it to Yourself

Avoid eating or drinking sugar or sugar substitutes for a month to see for yourself. It will probably be the most difficult month you have ever experienced. This is not an over-statement. Just try it. Not eating sugar in your diet for just three days will show you how difficult it is. Two weeks without sugar is like an alcoholic trying to quit drinking for the same period. What is really amusing, is that most reputable authorities think that sugar is not an addiction. But just try not eating sugar for two weeks and tell me that you are not addicted to sugar! I have been off sugar for years and I still CRAVE it. So don't think this will be easy.

The typical American diet includes a generous percentage of refined sugar. Sugar occurs naturally in many foods, such as fruit, which contains fructose. Trying to find food that you like, containing no sugar, is very difficult at first since you may not have given it much thought and especially if you eat a lot of processed food or eat in restaurants/fast food chains. Most processed food has sugar, as you will discover. However, you can still live a meaningful life without sugar. It can be done, many have done it, and you can too. I will tell you more on how you can get help avoiding sugar, and how to join *The Diet* Users Support Group for encouragement. But for now, just try to avoid eating sugar and carbohydrates for a month and eating a diet high in protein to see if your health gets better and if you lose weight.

During this one-month test, drink plenty of WATER. Please read the chapter on WATER.

Also, be sure to get enough VITAMINS in your diet, which will curb your appetite for sweets. Supplemental vitamins help so read the chapter on Vitamins and Supplements.

Get plenty of rest. If you are under a lot of stress, this will not help your diet, so don't add to your stress by overdoing it. Try to pick a thirty-day period that is stress free. Don't start this diet if you are under stress. The ideal thirty-day period to begin this diet is a long vacation. But even if you do not have the luxury to

50

avoid stress, you will find that to the extent you avoid sugar in your diet, you should notice some commensurate improvement in your health and some weight loss.

Exercise is necessary. You know all the authorities say exercise is needed for health. As *Newsweek*[1] puts it,

> "Diet alone, however, isn't enough. You also need to get moving. That doesn't mean you have to become an exercise maniac. A half-hour of brisk walking a day can dramatically lower your risk of chronic disease. The payoff for all this effort is huge: a longer, healthier life."

You know this is true. At the very least go on regular walks. Finding the time, motivation and will power to do this and to change your diet is the issue.

---

1.   *Newsweek*, January 20, 2003, p.45

Motivation and Will Power

What I have discovered is that those who say *The Diet* has not helped them is because they did not reduce their carbohydrate intake to less than 30 grams a day. This is not always the case, but it is the number one reason. They simply cannot stick to a high protein diet. Why? The will power necessary to avoid sugar and carbohydrates for thirty days is tremendous. Another reason is they cheated occasionally or didn't reduce their sugar intake enough due to carelessness. Some sprinkle sugar substitutes into their food and drink thinking this is ok, but cannot tell that sugar has crept into their food or drink and did not detect it since their taste buds are not sugar sensitive and ate more than 30 grams of carbohydrates a day unknowingly. That is why I recommend no sugar substitutes for thirty days so you can detect sugar in your food and drink. <u>AFTER</u> the thirty days you can experiment with sugar substitutes, just like any thing else you want.

You might not be aware of how sugar gets into your diet. And remember this isn't a controlled study, it is simply your ability to avoid sugar, in all its forms, artificial refined sugar [sucrose] or natural sugar, whether it is sucrose, fructose, lactose, maltose, glucose, etc. Do you actually read the ingredients written on the package, bottle, can, or wrap that your food or drink contains? Even "sugarless" products sometimes contain other sources of sugar like brown sugar, fructose, corn syrup, honey, molasses, maltose, glucose, or some synonym for sugar. The food labels have all sorts of ways to hide sugar. The processed food manufacturers have found so many ways to keep some form of sugar in a product that you have to become a detective to find it. Absolutely no honey or maple syrup! And in order for you to be able to detect anything sweet in your food for thirty days, <u>please don't eat any sugar substitute</u> since you will not detect if sugar is still present in the food or drink you are consuming. I know this is hard, but your taste buds need to be sensitive to anything sweet and artificial sweeteners mask any sugar that may be present. <u>Avoiding sugar substitutes solves this problem for thirty days!</u> Does this take motivation and will power? Not many have either one, so you have to ask yourself if you as the *diet authority* can simply do this for thirty days? There is light at the end of this tunnel! It is only thirty days.

Reading the Nutrition Food Label

Nutrition Facts Label on any packaging lists **TOTAL CARBOHYDRATE**, and then lists under this "**Sugars**" and/or "**Sugar Alcohols**" and the total grams per serving. This is the where you find sugar in the ingredients, even if it is hidden in the list by some other name not mentioned in the list above. I keep finding new ones. So if you find any that I have not listed in the chapter, **Sugars to Avoid**, let me know so I can add it to the list. More information on this can be found at this url >

http://www.stanford.edu/group/ketodiet/cholabel.html

Also, watch out for "SUGAR FREE" or 'NO SUGAR ADDED!' This only means no sucrose or NO MORE SUGAR added since it usually CONTAINS some form of sugar hidden in the ingredients in a different form! An interesting link you may check is "The Sugar Free Hoax" > http://www.wilstar.net/sugarfree

The way the **Nutrition Facts Label** lists food is the order of amounts. The most listed first and the least listed last. So if the sugar word shows up near the first of the list the product is loaded with sugar! If the sugar word shows up in the list at all, avoid the product for thirty days. Learning to read this label will really improve your health and you will lose weight. The USDA has some helpful links if you still have questions about this label.
http://www.cfsan.fda.gov/label.html
http://www.nal.usda.gov/fnic/cgi-bin/nut_search.pl

If an item contains less than 1 gram of sugar or carbohydrate in a serving, for example, dextrose, the Nutrition Food Label will say Zero Carbohydrate. The dextrose is less than one gram per serving or unit. The Nutrition Facts Label is where you find the carbohydrate and sugar content in any food or drink. This is the best way to discover the carbohydrate or sugar content. The ingredient list can be misleading and the processed food industry is good at hiding sugar on ingredient lists and packaging statements. The one good thing the government health authorities did was requiring the Nutrition Facts Label to know the truth about a product. The list of ingredients can be helpful but the real information is found in the **Nutrition Facts Label**. An excellent book to count carbohydrate grams is, *Dr. Atkins' New Carbohydrate Gram Counter*, 1996, M. Evans and Company, Inc, New York, New York at this url along with other diet books > http://www.rosacea-diet/html/dietbooks.html

Alcohol

Are you aware that some beer and wine contain added sugar? Most alcohol contains high concentrations of sugar. Alcohol manufactures are not required to list the ingredients so you will never see it on a label. Alcohol is made mostly with sugar. Lots of it. Distilled spirits are made from lots of sugar and good wine has high amounts of fructose. Beer is loaded with maltose or adulterated with sucrose. <u>So for one month no alcohol</u>, period. After the thirty days, you can return to your favorite alcohol. Also, if you are an alcoholic you may find out during this 30-day period you have a problem with it by avoiding it.

Wine and Beer are the highest in sugar content, while the distilled spirits have fewer calories. AFTER the 30 day Diet Plan you may discover how much alcohol you can consume without weight gain and feel healthy. The sugar in alcohol is what you need to avoid for 30 days to lose weight and feel good. To give you an idea about the carbohydrate gram count in alcohol, 12 fl. oz. of regular beer contains 13.7 grams of carbohydrates, 12 fl. oz of table wine contains 14.7 grams of carbohydrates, while distilled spirits (hard liquors such as whisky, Scotch, vodka, bourbon, gin, etc,) ANY PROOF of 1 fl. oz contain only a trace of carbohydrates! So if you consume alcohol AFTER THE THIRTY DAYS beer and wine may increase your weight. The distilled spirits you may find may not increase weight. Moderation is the key for good health.

What you do with alcohol after the thirty days is your choice. It may be that alcohol is related to some health problems you are having and by not consuming alcohol for thirty days you may discover some relief.

Remember to avoid alcohol for thirty days. You can do it. At the end of the thirty days you can have that drink! Remember that you are the *diet authority.*

What to Say to Critics When You Diet

What happens usually when you go on a diet is a struggle emotionally within and without. To combat this struggle within is to have the motivation to either lose weight or feel healthy. You are reading this book to strengthen your resolve. You are collecting information. Your inner struggle is tough enough to deal with. Now what about the struggle from the outside?

Your friends, family and acquaintances discovering you are on the diet will offer all sorts of ideas and opinions. After all, they are *diet authorities*. And as I already pointed out diet is a very controversial subject and everyone knows what you should eat or drink. The problem is dealing with these outside influences could hinder your resolve and dampen your will power. Other major outside forces are the advertising media who tempt food or drink you have resolved within to avoid. People who could care less whether you are on a diet or not and don't like you may pose problems. And of course there are health authorities and professionals who have great influence on you. You should, of course discuss changing your diet with your physician. If you are an independent sort, you may not be bothered by any of these outside forces. However you may be influenced to a great deal by these outside influences more than you realize and that is what this chapter is all about so you can skip it if you are one tough cookie. I mean a soy cookie[1].

For example, you go to a family gathering and Mom has made a special apple pie and bought your favorite homemade ice cream. You explain that you are on a diet. Mom says, 'That's nice, here just have a little, I made this especially for you." You firm and refuse. You stand your ground and won't eat it. Your Mom's response turns into an emotional outburst. "YOU DON'T LOVE ME! You try

---

1.   www.puredeliteproducts.com
      Pure DeLite makes some sugar free products with maltitol one of which is a soy cookie

to explain, but nothing seems to change her mood. You finally give in because, after all, you do love your mother. This scene replays over and over with your mate, other family members and your friends. No matter how you explain your diet when it comes to eating with family and friends, food evokes emotional responses in everyone including you. Feelings are deeply rooted in what we eat and drink.

Remember the scene in the movie, *My Big Fat Greek Wedding*, when the star is trying to explain to her aunt that her fiancé is a vegetarian and the reaction of the family? The family is stunned! The aunt says, 'That's ok, I'll make lamb!"

Examples like this are repeated over and over when you tell anyone that you are on a diet and can't eat apple pie or ice cream. Emotional responses like 'What is wrong with apple pie and ice cream? You might as well tell me that John Wayne burned an American flag!'

There is absolutely no way to reasonably respond to emotion. Logic doesn't work. No explanation will change the feeling. Usually you respond with more emotion. What can you do?

Understanding the emotional feelings that are deeply rooted in eating and drinking with friends and family will help you to be better able to cope with these situations. You can assure your friends and family of your love. Explain that this diet is only for thirty days and mention what number day you are on and how many more are left. You may take them up on the food or drink offered when the thirty days are up. This may appease your well-intentioned friends and family. You may come up with a better plan than this. Just remember that during the thirty days you may have many friends, family members or whomever try to pressure you into eating and drinking sugar and carbohydrate. When this happens you must be mentally and emotionally prepared what you will say. I have given you some suggested statements to make and you may even come up with some better ones. Your suggestions are welcome and may be posted at *The Diet* Users Support Group at yahoo groups, which is the subject of another chapter.

When discussing this diet with your health care provider it would be wise to advise the practitioner that this diet is for only thirty days and that there are no known health risks of altering your diet for thirty days. Explain that this diet is approximately 64% protein, 30% fat, and 6% carbohydrate for just thirty days.

Most professional health care providers will not object to such a diet for such a short period. After the thirty days you may eat whatever you want.

How Can I Get Additional Suport?

Join **The Diet Users Support Group** at yahoo groups by sending an email to this address:

the-diet-users-support-group-subscribe@yahoogroups.com

If you join *Diet* Users Support Group there is a database of **recipes** available. There are links to related web sites to check but another chapter explains about this group with detailed information.

Also there are five books which I recommend as additional reading which will actually help you and may change your eating habits for life! Here is the list:

Sugar Blues by William Dufty, 175, Warner Books, Inc
Sugar Busters! By H. Leighton Steward, Dr. Morrison C. Bethea, Dr. Samuel S. Andrews, and Dr. Luis A Balart, 15, *Sugar Busters!*, LLC
Protein Power by Michael R. Eades, M.D. and Mary Dan Eades, M.D., 16, Bantam Books
Dr. Atkins' New Carbohydrate Gram Counter by Robert C. Atkins, 1996, M.D., M. Evans and Company, Inc
Dr. Atkin's New Diet Revolution by Robert C. Atkins, M.D., 2001, Avon

These books will verify the need to find a diet avoiding sugar in all its forms. Like I said, this isn't going to be easy, especially if you eat out a lot. You may need additional support. You already know that all the food you eat is eventually converted to glucose so your cells can use the energy from what you eat. Your body takes a lot more time and energy to convert protein to glucose through protein synthesis, which is discussed in another chapter. By reading these books you will also discover a lot of information which will help you understand the role insulin and glucagon has on your body. Glucagon is a hormone secreted by the pancreas that helps regulate blood sugar and metabolize stored fat. Could it be possible that eating sugar over the years taxes the pancreas upsetting the hormonal balance in our immune system and we need to stimulate glucagon in our bodies to get healthy? Insulin dominance in our body as a result of eating too much sugar in the diet over the years should be replaced with a glucagon dominance in our body by avoiding sugar and eating a high protein diet. Could it be that sugar is just a poison that over many years of consumption causes vascular disorders or cancers? Mr. Dufty, in *Sugar Blues* did not discuss the role glucagon has on the body when he wrote his book in 1975, and didn't understand that a diet high in protein is preferable, but instead encouraged a diet high in carbohydrates, which has been popular for years. Dufty's diet, or a high carbohydrate diet will increase blood glucose levels, so I recommend the diet mentioned in *Protein Power* as my preference, but the diet in *Sugar Busters!* is useful. However, Mr. Dufty's book on sugar is the premier source of information on the history of sugar, its sordid past and its unhealthy effects, including the sugar blues. All five books are currently available and can easily be obtained by going online to this site:

http://rosacea-control.com/html/dietbooks.html

You will also find on this web page some other suggested diet books that will help you find recipes avoiding sugar and carbohydrates to help you. As I said, there are thousands of diet books out there, but I have selected some that are in harmony with *The Diet* and you might find some interesting reading.

Ten Suggestions for the Thirty Day Diet Plan

1. Do not eat sugar, sucrose, maltose, lactose, glucose, fructose, or sugar substitutes such as saccharin, cyclamates, aspartame, acesulfame-K or any natural sugar substitute, just for thirty days—See the chapter **Sugars to Avoid.**

2. Do not eat carbohydrate or starches unless specifically mentioned in the 30-Day *Diet* Plan—Limit your total carbohydrate intake to 30 grams or less! Read the Nutrition Facts Label on all foods and drinks to determine carbohydrate gram content and **DO NOT EXCEED 30 GRAMS PER DAY!**
An excellent source for counting carbohydrate grams is found in the chapter on **Reading the Nutrition Label.**

3. Do not smoke or use tobacco[1] for thirty days

4. Drink EIGHT 12 oz. glasses of water every day (TEN glasses are recommended)

5. Take plenty of vitamins—see chapter on **Vitamin & Mineral Supplements**

6. Get plenty of rest and sleep

7. Do not consume ANY ALCOHOL for 30 days—see chapter on **Alcohol**

8. Always remember this is a 30-day test to see if you lose weight or feel healthier, remember, this is a test—at the end of the thirty days you can return to eating whatever you want!

---

1. **"an average of 5 percent sugar is added to cigarettes**, up to 20 per cent in cigars, and as much as 40 per cent in pipe tobacco, mostly in the form of molasses and such…flue-cured tobacco can contain as much as 20 percent sugar by weight…sugar (sucrose) is added to air-cured tobacco during the blending process…"—from *Sugar Blues* by William Dufty, 1975 Warner Books, p.190, 192

9. Do not cheat

10. Eat protein, protein, **PROTEIN, as much as you want,** and don't worry about any of the fat that comes with the protein—You won't go hungry on this diet since you can eat all the protein you want!

30 Days—30 Grams of Carbohydrates a Day—No Sugar

The Diet 30-Day Diet Plan is for only thirty days. After you have proven to yourself that this diet works, you can then eat whatever you want, or modify this diet any way you think best. *The Diet* is simply the beginning of a new life style diet that works for you. Go ahead and eat all those sugar delights you crave and see if your weight returns or your health diminishes. If you wish to control your weight or feel healthier, you can go back on *The Diet* or modify it any way you want with additional carbohydrates till you find the diet you can control your control your weight or feel healthy with your eating habits. Remember the 8th suggestion, "Always remember this is a 30 day test to see if this controls your weight and feel healthier, remember, this is a test." If the test proves true, you can then decide for yourself how you are going to control your weight and feel healthy with your diet any way you want after the test.

You should eat less than 30 grams of carbohydrates a day during the thirty day *Diet Plan*. If you eat more than 30 grams of carbohydrates per day, your weight may remain the same. You need to learn how to count your carbs! Once source is *Sugar Busters!* which is an excellent source for counting carbs and understanding the glycemic index, which is discussed in a later chapter. 30 days, 30 grams of carbohydrates and NO SUGAR of any kind.

By the way when you eat salt, be sure to check the box of salt and see if DEXTROSE is added to your salt. I suggest sea salt or at the very least kosher salt. Sea Salt is better for you than the processed salt with dextrose added. Even if you find processed salt without dextrose or sugar it is still refined so much that all the essential minerals are removed. If you do a search on sea salt or the brand Celtic Salt you will find some interesting information why sea salt is better than the processed salt with or without dextrose. One url to consider is >

http://www.elementsofwellness.com/celticsalt.htm

There are other sites that discuss the advantages of sea salt over processed table salt which has all the minerals removed that your body needs. Did you know that salt is an essential element the body needs and yet the health authorities have made salt just as evil as fat? Why would they make salt, an essential mineral, a bad guy?

Thirty Day Meat Eaters Diet Plan

The next thirty days will prove whether you can control your weight and feel healthier with your diet if you stick to this diet and don't cheat! The good thing about this diet is that you can eat as much as you want of the proteins listed each day! You just have to limit your carbohydrates to 30 grams a day. All you have to do is avoid any sugar, syrups, honey, sugar substitutes, carbohydrates, starches, breads, grains, or fruits not specifically mentioned in the diet. And NO tobacco, because sugar is in your tobacco. Your total carbohydrate intake for EACH day should be 30 grams or less during this thirty day *Diet* plan [remember the Second Suggestion].

No matter if you are a vegetarian or a meat eater, avoid raisins, bananas, all fruits, fruit juices, parsnips, honey, carrots, corn/cornflakes, millet, beets, white rice, pasta, plain crackers, all types of white flour, or any potatoes (any color). All these foods easily convert to glucose and should be avoided for thirty days.

Meat eaters should **AVOID ALL GRAINS** for the thirty-day diet plan. After the thirty days, you can eat as much grain as you want. Grain, of course, includes all bread, pasta, etc., which have too many carbohydrate grams during this thirty-day period. AFTER the thirty days, you can begin experimenting with grains to see your weight return or health problems come back.

Eating just a small amount of catsup, or chocolate, or tablespoon of ice cream is cheating! That nice juicy apple is loaded with fructose, so don't cheat! If your weight is obese, it will take a month or more before you notice any improvement. But stick to the Thirty-Day *Diet* Plan and see the results for yourself.

Nuts are acceptable for snacks, peanuts being the first choice, which contain 5 grams carbs), but other nuts may be better for health, so I recommend mixed nuts containing NO PEANUTS. If you have no issues with peanuts, go ahead and eat them but count the carbohydrate gram content and include this in the total for the day. Eat no more than 30 grams of carbohydrate a day including the peanuts! Peanuts may produce an allergy in you if you eat too many so be fore-warned. It is possible that you may have a peanut allergy check this web site:

http://www.skincarecampaign.org/peanutall.htm

So you better be careful with peanuts. I have found that mixed nuts containing NO PEANUTS work better for me but during this 30-day period you have to keep your nuts to a minimum. For example, 3 tablespoons of mixed nuts without peanuts (or 28 grams) contain 7 grams of carbohydrates. You can only eat 30 grams of carbohydrates a day. Don't go nuts! If you have to have something sweet, the only fruit allowed to eat is avocados and grapefruits, which aren't sweet, so if you have to, I allow dried apricots, but don't eat more than TWO BITES a day! Two halves of dried apricots contain 5 grams carbs. I have found that sugar substitutes should be avoided during this thirty-day diet plan.

Snacks that you can substitute during the 30-day test are as follows:
Nuts, sunflower seeds, pork rinds, lean meat slices, any cheese, almond butter without sugar, celery with cream cheese, dried apricot slices, jerky containing no sugar, hard boiled egg, peanut butter without sugar, WASA Original Crispbread Light Rye (each cracker is 6 grams of carbohydrate/1 Gram Protein). I prefer Ryvita crackers over WASA. Remember to count the total grams per day of car-bohydrates of your snacks and meals to 30 grams or less per day as I have men-tioned many times. Another crispbread that you might like better is Ryvita.

Your total carbohydrate intake per day should not exceed 30 grams, including snacks. Count those carbs! Eat as much protein as you want and don't worry about any of the fat during this 30-day period. Remember that this is only for 30 days to see if you can lose weight and feel healthy.

During the thirty days you may substitute a protein (i.e. meat, fish, chicken) with another protein. You can modify it to fit your situation. The thirty-day sugges-tions will give you an idea of how to reduce your carbohydrates to 30 grams a day and eat AS MUCH PROTEIN AS YOU WANT. Yes, I said you could eat as much protein as you want. You just limit the carbohydrates to 30 grams a day. You may substitute a carbohydrate with another carbohydrate as long as you keep within the 30-gram limit per day.

No sugar in sausage which may not be easy to find, but try to find it. If you can-not find sugarless sausage, substitute sugarless bacon, which usually is easier to obtain. By the way, after the 30 days, you may be able to tolerate bacon, sausage or ham whether it is sugar cured or not, you will just have to experiment. But during the thirty days of the diet, do not eat sugar-cured bacon, sausage, ham, or any sugar-cured meat.

You may add heavy cream to the black coffee or tea during the thirty-day diet whether you are a meat eater or vegetarian. Do not use half-and-half or milk since there is carbohydrate in milk or half-and-half and none in heavy cream. You will enjoy the heavy cream more. The reason I put black coffee is so you don't think you can add any Creamora or any cream substitute because such products are loaded with sugar or sugar substitute.

Meat eaters complain that the thirty-day diet plan includes expensive cuts of meats. Remember that this is for just thirty days. After the thirty days you can save all the money you want. Usually you eat out in fast food restaurants or you may even go to expensive restaurants and think nothing of the bill. If you could sacrifice eating out for one month I think that should easily cover the extra cost of the expensive cuts of meats. How much do you spend on your bar bill or the liquor store a month? If you follow my suggestions you will save on junk food, sugar items, desserts, pastries, liquor and many other sugar products. The savings from avoiding these products for a month more than off sets the expensive meats. But of course, you may substitute the expensive cuts of meats with the inexpensive cuts. So don't get all excited when you see an expensive cut of meat on the diet, since you as the diet authority may substitute the expensive cut with an inexpensive one. If you substitute carbohydrates, just be sure to stay with the 30 grams a day limit.

Day One	Meat Eaters Menu Anyone may Eat as much protein as you want! SUBSTITUTE any PROTEIN with a Protein	Carbohydrate Grams Just Limit your Carbohydrates To 30 Grams per day!
breakfast	at wake up—12 oz. glass of water, Sausage and eggs, salt, one cup black coffee or tea, 12 oz glass of water, vitamins	Zero carbs
Break	12 oz glass of water, cheese	5 oz of cheddar—3 grams carbs
Lunch	12 oz glass of water, half avocado with tuna, chicken, or crab with vinegar & oil, chopped hard-boiled egg with fresh salad greens, black olives, tomato (vinegar and oil) one cup black coffee or tea, 12 oz glass of water	half Florida avocado— 6.5 grams carbs 1 cup of salad greens— 2 grams carbs Half tomato—3 grams carbs
Break	12 oz glass of water, cheese	5 oz of cheddar—3 grams carbs
Supper	12 oz glass of water, Beef tenderloin (or other lean cut) asparagus spears with cheese, fresh green salad (vinegar and oil) tea, 12 oz. glass of water	4 asparagus spears— 2.2 grams carbs 5 oz cheese—3 grams carbs 1 cup of salad—2 grams carbs
Day One	Before bed 12 oz glass of water, if you wake up in the night, drink 12 oz glass of water	Total carbohydrates = Less than 30 grams carbs

	Meat Eaters Menu Anyone may Eat as much protein as you want! SUBSTITUTE any PROTEIN with a Protein	Carbohydrate Grams Just Limit your Carbohydrates to 30 grams per day!
Day Two		
breakfast	at wake up—12 oz. glass of water, Bacon [not sugar cured] and eggs, salt one cup black coffee or tea, 12 oz glass of water, vitamins	Zero carbs
Break	12 oz glass of water, cheese	5 oz of cheddar—3 grams carbs
Lunch	12 oz glass of water, pork chops, cottage cheese fresh green salad (vinegar and oil) with tomato one cup black coffee or tea, 12 oz glass of water	1 cup whole milk cottage cheese —8 grams carbs 1 cup of salad greens— 2 grams carbs Half tomato—3 grams carbs
Break	12 oz glass of water, cheese (your choice)	5 oz of cheddar—3 grams carbs
Supper	12 oz glass of water, meat loaf (no sugar, syrup, catsup, raisins, carrots in meatloaf) cabbage cole slaw or fresh green salad (vinegar and oil) 12 oz glass of water, tea	Half cup cole slaw w/dressing —4.25 grams carbs or 1 cup of salad greens— 2 grams carbs
Day Two	Before bed 12 oz glass of water, if you wake up in the night, drink 12 oz glass of water	Total carbohydrates = Less than 30 grams carbs

Day Three	Meat Eaters Menu Anyone may Eat as much protein as you want! SUBSTITUTE any PROTEIN with a Protein	Carbohydrate Grams Just Limit your Carbohydrates to 30 grams per day!
breakfast	at wake up—12 oz. glass of water, cheese omelet, salt, one cup black coffee or tea 12 oz glass of water, vitamins	5 oz. cheese in omelet— 3 grams carbs
break	12 oz glass of water, nuts with celery	1 tablespoon mixed nuts— 2 grams carbs 2 stalks celery—3 grams carbs
Lunch	12 oz glass of water, chicken, Cole slaw (no sugar in dressing) or fresh green salad (vinegar and oil) one cup black coffee or tea 12 oz glass of water	Half cup cole slaw w/dressing —4.25 grams carbs or 1 cup of salad greens— 2 grams carbs
Break	12 oz glass of water, nuts with celery	1 tablespoon mixed nuts— 2 grams carbs 2 stalks celery—3 grams carbs
Supper	12 oz glass of water, meat loaf (no sugar, syrup, catsup, raisins, carrots in meatloaf) cabbage cole slaw, fresh green salad (vinegar and oil) 12 oz glass of water, tea	Half cup cole slaw w/dressing —4.25 grams carbs 1 cup of salad greens— 2 grams carbs
Day Three	Before bed 12 oz glass of water, if you wake up in the night, drink 12 oz glass of water	Total carbohydrates = Less than 30 grams carbs

Day Four	**Meat Eaters Menu** Anyone may Eat as much protein as you want! SUBSTITUTE any PROTEIN with a Protein	**Carbohydrate Grams** Just Limit your Carbohydrates to 30 grams per day!
breakfast	at wake up—12 oz. glass of water, Bacon [not sugar cured] and eggs, salt, one cup black coffee or tea, 12 oz glass of water, vitamins	Zero carbs
Break	12 oz glass of water, cheese	5 oz cheese—3 grams carbs
Lunch	12 oz glass of water, fish, half avocado and peppers green salad (vinegar and oil) one cup black coffee or tea 12 oz glass of water	Half Calif. Avocado— 6.5 grams carbs Half cup green pepper— 3 grams carbs 1 cup of salad greens— 2 grams carbs
Break	12 oz glass of water, cheese	5 oz cheese—3 grams carbs
Supper	12 oz glass of water, corned beef and cabbage, fresh green salad (vinegar and oil) 12 oz glass of water, tea	1 cup cooked cabbage— 6 grams carbs 1 cup of salad greens— 2 grams carbs
Day Four	Before bed 12 oz glass of water, if you wake up in the night, drink 12 oz glass of water	Total carbohydrates = Less than 30 grams carbs

Day Five	**Meat Eaters Menu** Anyone may Eat as much protein as you want! SUBSTITUTE any PROTEIN with a Protein	**Carbohydrate Grams** Just Limit your Carbohydrates to 30 grams per day!
breakfast	at wake up—12 oz. glass of water, Canadian bacon [not sugar cured] & eggs, salt, one cup black coffee or tea, 12 oz glass of water, vitamins	Trace carbs in Canadian Bacon
Break	12 oz glass of water, cheese and nuts	5 oz cheese—3 grams carbs 2 tablespoons of Mixed nuts—3.5 grams carbs
Lunch	12 oz glass of water, hamburger patty and cottage cheese fresh green salad (vinegar and oil) one cup black coffee or tea 12 oz glass of water	One cup of whole milk cottage cheese—8 grams carbs 1 cup of salad greens—2 grams carbs
Break	12 oz glass of water, celery with cream cheese and nuts	tablespoons cream cheese—2 grams carbs 2 stalks celery—3.2 grams carbs 1 tablespoon mixed nuts—2.3 grams carbs
Supper	12 oz glass of water, chef salad with meat (vinegar and oil) 12 oz glass of water, tea	Chef salad—5 grams carbs estimated
Day Five	Before bed 12 oz glass of water, if you wake up in the night, drink 12 oz glass of water	Total carbohydrates = around 30 grams carbs

Day Six	**Meat Eaters Menu** Anyone may Eat as much protein as you want! SUBSTITUTE any PROTEIN with a Protein	**Carbohydrate Grams** Just Limit your Carbohydrates to 30 grams per day!
breakfast	at wake up—12 oz. glass of water, steak & eggs, salt, one cup black coffee or tea, 12 oz glass of water, vitamins	Zero carbs
Break	12 oz glass of water, cheese and nuts	5 oz cheese—3 grams carbs 2 tablespoons of Mixed nuts—4.6 grams carbs
Lunch	12 oz glass of water, fish with tofu or spinach fresh green salad (vinegar and oil) one cup black coffee or tea 12 oz glass of water	One cup cooked spinach—6.5 grams carbs 1 cup of salad greens—2 grams carbs
Break	12 oz glass of water, celery with cream cheese and nuts	4 tablespoons cream cheese—2 grams carbs 2 stalks celery—3.2 grams carbs
Supper	12 oz glass of water, cheeseburger patty and eggplant fresh green salad (vinegar and oil) 12 oz glass of water	Half cup eggplant—4.1 grams carbs 1 cup of salad greens—2 grams carbs
Day Six	Before bed 12 oz glass of water, if you wake up in the night, drink 12 oz glass of water	Total carbohydrates = less than 30 grams carbs

Day Seven	Meat Eaters Menu Anyone may Eat as much protein as you want! SUBSTITUTE any PROTEIN with a Protein	Carbohydrate Grams Just Limit your Carbohydrates to 30 grams per day!
breakfast	at wake up—12 oz. glass of water, tofu or eggs and cottage cheese one cup black coffee or tea, 12 oz glass of water, vitamins	Half cup whole milk cottage cheese—4 grams carbs 2 in. cube tofu—2.9 grams carbs
Break	12 oz glass of water, two hard boiled eggs	zero carbs
Lunch	12 oz glass of water, fish and peppers, broccoli, OR green beans fresh green salad (vinegar and oil) one cup black coffee or tea 12 oz glass of water	Half cup diced peppers— 3 grams carbs Half cup broccoli—4 grams carbs Half cup green snap beans— 3.4 grams carbs 1 cup of salad greens— 2 grams carbs
Break	12 oz glass of water, celery with cream cheese and nuts	2 tablespoons cream cheese— 1 grams carbs 2 stalks celery—3.2 grams carbs 1 tablespoons mixed nuts— 2 grams carbs
Supper	12 oz glass of water, steak and asparagus, salt, fresh green salad (vinegar and oil) 12 oz glass of water	4 asparagus spears— 2.2 grams carbs 1 cup of salad greens— 2 grams carbs
Day Seven	Before bed 12 oz glass of water, if you wake up in the night, drink 12 oz glass of water	Total carbohydrates = less than 30 grams carbs

	Meat Eaters Menu Anyone may Eat as much protein as you want! SUBSTITUTE any PROTEIN with a Protein	Carbohydrate Grams Just Limit your Carbohydrates to 30 grams per day!
Day Eight		
breakfast	at wake up—12 oz. glass of water, cheese omelet with celery and peppers one cup black coffee or tea 12 oz glass of water, vitamins	2 oz cheese—1.2 grams carbs 1 stalk celery—1.6 grams carbs Quarter cup green peppers—2.5 grams carbs
Break	12 oz glass of water, cheese and nuts	2 oz cheese—1.2 grams carbs One and half tablespoons of mixed nuts—3.5 grams carbs
Lunch	12 oz glass of water, steak and eggs fresh green salad (vinegar and oil) one cup black coffee or tea 12 oz glass of water	1 cup of salad greens—2 grams carbs
Break	12 oz glass of water, celery with cream cheese and nuts	2 tablespoons cream cheese—1 grams carbs 2 stalks celery—3.2 grams carbs One and half tablespoons of mixed nuts—3.5 grams carbs
Supper	12 oz glass of water, fish with cucumbers, mushrooms, peppers fresh green salad (vinegar and oil) 12 oz glass of water	Half cucumber—1.8 grams carbs Half cup mushrooms—2.6 grams carbs Half cup green pepper—3.6 grams carbs 1 cup of salad greens—2 grams carbs
Day Eight	Before bed 12 oz glass of water, if you wake up in the night, drink 12 oz glass of water	Total carbohydrates = around 30 grams carbs

Day Nine	Meat Eaters Menu Anyone may Eat as much protein as you want! SUBSTITUTE any PROTEIN with a Protein	Carbohydrate Grams Just Limit your Carbohydrates to 30 grams per day!
breakfast	at wake up—12 oz. glass of water, steak and eggs, salt, one cup black coffee or tea, 12 oz glass of water, vitamins	zero carbs
Break	12 oz glass of water, cheese and nuts 3 oz cheese	5 oz cheese—3 grams carbs Three tablespoons of mixed nuts—7 grams carbs
Lunch	12 oz glass of water, fish and green peppers, fresh green salad (vinegar and oil) one cup black coffee or tea 12 oz glass of water	One pepper—7.2 grams carbs 1 cup of salad greens— 2 grams carbs
Break	12 oz glass of water, two hard boiled eggs, nuts	One and half tablespoons of mixed nuts—3.5 grams carbs
Supper	12 oz glass of water, chef salad with meat (vinegar and oil) 12 oz glass of water, tea	chef salad— 5 grams carbs estimated
Day Nine	Before bed 12 oz glass of water, if you wake up in the night, drink 12 oz glass of water	Total carbohydrates = less than 30 grams carbs

Day Ten	Meat Eaters Menu Anyone may Eat as much protein as you want! SUBSTITUTE any PROTEIN with a Protein	Carbohydrate Grams Just Limit your Carbohydrates to 30 grams per day!
breakfast	at wake up—12 oz. glass of water, sausage and eggs one cup black coffee or tea, 12 oz glass of water, vitamins	zero carbs
Break	12 oz glass of water, cheese and nuts	3 oz cheese—1.8 grams carbs One and half tablespoons of mixed nuts—3.5 grams carbs
Lunch	12 oz glass of water, cheeseburger patty and cottage cheese fresh green salad (vinegar and oil) one cup black coffee or tea 12 oz glass of water	2 oz cheese—1.2 grams carbs 1 cup of salad greens—2 grams carbs
Break	12 oz glass of water, celery with cream cheese and nuts	2 stalks celery—3.2 grams carbs 2 tablespoons cream cheese—2 grams carbs 3 tablespoons mixed nuts—7 grams carbs
Supper	12 oz glass of water, steak with mushrooms, zucchini, spinach fresh green salad (vinegar and oil) 12 oz glass of water	Half cup mushrooms—1.5 grams carbs Half cup zucchini—2.6 grams carbs 1 cup raw spinach—2.4 grams carbs
Day Ten	Before bed 12 oz glass of water, if you wake up in the night, drink 12 oz glass of water	Total carbohydrates = less than 30 grams carbs

Day Eleven	Meat Eaters Menu Anyone may Eat as much protein as you want! SUBSTITUTE any PROTEIN with a Protein	Carbohydrate Grams Just Limit your Carbohydrates to 30 grams per day!
breakfast	at wake up—12 oz. glass of water, cheese omelet with cottage cheese one cup black coffee or tea, 12 oz glass of water, vitamins	3 oz cheese—1.2 grams carbs Half cup whole milk cottage cheese—4 grams carbs
Break	12 oz glass of water, celery with cream cheese and nuts	3 stalks celery—4.8 grams carbs 3 tablespoons cream cheese—1.5 grams carbs One and half tablespoons of mixed nuts—3.5 grams carbs
Lunch	12 oz glass of water, pork chops and green beans, fresh green salad (vinegar and oil), one cup black coffee or tea, 12 oz glass of water	Half cup snap green beans—3.4 grams carb 1 cup of salad greens—2 grams carbs
Break	12 oz glass of water, two hard boiled eggs	zero carbs
Supper	12 oz glass of water, chicken with spinach, fresh green salad (vinegar and oil) 12 oz glass of water, tea	One cup cooked spinach—6.5 grams carbs 1 cup of salad greens—2 grams carbs
Day Eleven	Before bed 12 oz glass of water, if you wake up in the night, drink 12 oz glass of water	Total carbohydrates = less than 30 grams carbs

Day Twelve	Meat Eaters Menu Anyone may Eat as much protein as you want! SUBSTITUTE any PROTEIN with a Protein	Carbohydrate Grams Just Limit your Carbohydrates to 30 grams per day!
breakfast	at wake up—12 oz. glass of water, bacon [not sugar cured] and eggs, salt, one cup black coffee or tea, 12 oz glass of water, vitamins	zero carbs
Break	12 oz glass of water, celery with almond butter	2 stalks celery—3.2 grams carbs Quarter oz almond butter—3.6 grams carbs
Lunch	12 oz glass of water, salmon with broccoli, fresh green salad (vinegar and oil) one cup black coffee or tea 12 oz glass of water	Half cup broccoli—4.25 grams/carb 1 cup of salad greens—2 grams carbs
Break	12 oz glass of water, celery with cream cheese and nuts	3 stalks celery—4 .8 grams carbs 3 tablespoons cream cheese—1.5 grams carbs One and half tablespoons of mixed nuts—3.5 grams carbs
Supper	12 oz glass of water, Pork loin with asparagus/melted cheese fresh green salad (vinegar and oil) 12 oz glass of water, tea	1 oz cheese—.6 gram/carb 8 asparagus spears—4.4 grams carbs 1 cup of salad greens—2 grams carbs
Day Twelve	Before bed 12 oz glass of water, if you wake up in the night, drink 12 oz glass of water	Total carbohydrates = less than 30 grams carbs

Day Thirteen	Meat Eaters Menu Anyone may Eat as much protein as you want! SUBSTITUTE any PROTEIN with a Protein	Carbohydrate Grams Just Limit your Carbohydrates to 30 grams per day!
breakfast	at wake up—12 oz. glass of water, eggs and sausage, salt, one cup black coffee or tea, 12 oz glass of water, vitamins	zero carbs
Break	12 oz glass of water, celery with cream cheese and nuts	2 stalks celery—3.2 grams carbs 3 tablespoons cream cheese—1.5 grams carbs One and half tablespoons of mixed nuts—3.5 grams carbs
Lunch	12 oz glass of water, steak with egg-plant, fresh green salad (vinegar and oil) one cup black coffee or tea 12 oz glass of water	Half cup eggplant—4.1 grams carb 1 cup of salad greens—2 grams carbs
Break	12 oz glass of water, cheese and nuts	3 oz cheese—1.8 grams carbs One and half tablespoons of mixed nuts—3.5 grams carbs
Supper	12 oz glass of water, prime roast beef with mushrooms and green beans fresh green salad (vinegar and oil) 12 oz glass of water, tea	Half cup mushrooms—2.5 gram carb Half cup snap green beans—3.4 grams carbs 1 cup of salad greens—2 grams carbs
Day Thirteen	Before bed 12 oz glass of water, if you wake up in the night, drink 12 oz glass of water	Total carbohydrates = less than 30 grams carbs

Day Fourteen	Meat Eaters Menu Anyone may Eat as much protein as you want! SUBSTITUTE any PROTEIN with a Protein	Carbohydrate Grams Just Limit your Carbohydrates to 30 grams per day!
breakfast	at wake up—12 oz. glass of water, cheese omelet with celery and peppers. one cup black coffee or tea, 12 oz glass of water, vitamins	1 oz. cheese—.6 grams carbs 1 stalk celery—1.6 grams carbs Half cup green pepper—3.4 grams carbs
Break	12 oz glass of water, nuts	3 tablespoons of mixed nuts—7 grams carbs
Lunch	12 oz glass of water, cheeseburger patty with mushrooms fresh green salad (vinegar and oil) one cup black coffee or tea 12 oz glass of water	Half cup eggplant—4.1 grams carb 1 cup of salad greens—2 grams carbs
Break	12 oz glass of water, celery with cream cheese	3 stalks celery—4.8 grams carbs 3 tablespoons cream cheese—1.5 grams carbs
Supper	12 oz glass of water, fillet mignon and mushrooms fresh green salad (vinegar and oil) 12 oz glass of water, tea	Half cup mushrooms—2.5 gram carb 1 cup of salad greens—2 grams carbs
Day Fourteen	Before bed 12 oz glass of water, if you wake up in the night, drink 12 oz glass of water	Total carbohydrates = less than 30 grams carbs

Day Fifteen	Meat Eaters Menu Anyone may Eat as much protein as you want! SUBSTITUTE any PROTEIN with a Protein	Carbohydrate Grams Just Limit your Carbohydrates to 30 grams per day!
breakfast	at wake up—12 oz. glass of water, Ham and eggs, one cup black coffee, or tea, 12 oz glass of water, vitamins	zero carbs
Break	12 oz glass of water, nuts	3 tablespoons of mixed nuts—7 grams carbs
Lunch	12 oz glass of water, fish or seafood [no batter] spinach, fresh green salad with vinegar and oil, one cup black coffee or tea 12 oz glass of water	1 cup spinach—6.5 grams carb 1 cup of salad greens—2 grams carbs
Break	12 oz glass of water, celery with cream cheese	3 stalks celery—4.8 grams carbs 3 tablespoons cream cheese—1.5 grams carbs
Supper	12 oz glass of water, Pork or Lamb, scallions, peppers, and fresh lettuce, grape tomatoes with vinegar and oil 12 oz glass of water, tea	2 tablespoons scallions—2 grams carbs 1 cup of salad greens—2 grams carbs 5 grape tomatoes—3 grams carbs
Day Fifteen	Before bed 12 oz glass of water, if you wake up in the night, drink 12 oz glass of water	Total carbohydrates = less than 30 grams carbs

Day Sixteen	Meat Eaters Menu Anyone may Eat as much protein as you want! SUBSTITUTE any PROTEIN with a Protein	Carbohydrate Grams Just Limit your Carbohydrates to 30 grams per day!
breakfast	at wake up—12 oz. glass of water, Steak and eggs, salt, one cup black coffee, or tea 12 oz glass of water, vitamins	zero carbs
Break	12 oz glass of water, nuts	3 tablespoons of mixed nuts— 7 grams carbs
Lunch	12 oz glass of water, cheeseburger patty with mushrooms fresh green salad (vinegar and oil) one cup black coffee or tea 12 oz glass of water	1 oz cheese—.6 grams carb 1 cup of salad greens— 2 grams carbs
Break	12 oz glass of water, two hard boiled eggs	zero carbs
Supper	12 oz glass of water, fish or seafood [no batter], collard greens, fresh green salad with vinegar and oil, one cup black coffee or tea 12 oz glass of water	1 cup collard greens— 9.8 grams carbs 1 cup of salad greens— 2 grams carbs 5 grape tomatoes— 3 grams carbs
Day Sixteen	Before bed 12 oz glass of water, if you wake up in the night, drink 12 oz glass of water	Total carbohydrates = less than 30 grams carbs

Day Seventeen	Meat Eaters Menu Anyone may Eat as much protein as you want! SUBSTITUTE any PROTEIN with a Protein	Carbohydrate Grams Just Limit your Carbohydrates to 30 grams per day!
breakfast	at wake up—12 oz. glass of water, bacon [not sugar cured] and eggs with one cup black coffee, or tea, 12 oz glass of water, vitamins	zero carbs
Break	12 oz glass of water, nuts	3 tablespoons of mixed nuts—7 grams carbs
Lunch	12 oz glass of water, salmon with salsa, asparagus spears & butter fresh green salad (vinegar and oil) one cup black coffee or tea 12 oz glass of water	2 tablespoons salsa—2.5 grams carbs 4 asparagus spears—2.2 grams carbs 1 cup of salad greens—2 grams carbs
Break	12 oz glass of water, celery with cream cheese	2 stalks celery—3.2 grams carbs 2 tablespoons cream cheese—1 grams carbs
Supper	12 oz glass of water, baked ham [salt cured, not sugar cured] and collard greens fresh green salad (vinegar and oil) 12 oz glass of water, tea	1 cup collard greens—9.8 grams carbs 1 cup of salad greens—2 grams carbs
Day Seventeen	Before bed 12 oz glass of water, if you wake up in the night, drink 12 oz glass of water	Total carbohydrates = less than 30 grams carbs

Day Eighteen	Meat Eaters Menu Anyone may Eat as much protein as you want! SUBSTITUTE any PROTEIN with a Protein	Carbohydrate Grams Just Limit your Carbohydrates to 30 grams per day!
breakfast	at wake up—12 oz. glass of water, Spanish omelet, salt, one cup black coffee, or tea, 12 oz glass of water, vitamins	Half cup green peppers—3.6 grams carbs Half tomato—3 grams carbs Quarter cup onions—3.7 grams carbs 1 oz cheese—.6 gram/carb
Break	12 oz glass of water, celery	3 celery stalks—4.8 grams carbs
Lunch	12 oz glass of water, chicken, turnip, fresh green salad with vinegar and oil, one cup black coffee or tea 12 oz glass of water	Half turnip—4.3 grams carbs 1 cup of salad greens—2 grams carbs
Break	12 oz glass of water, two hard boiled eggs	zero carbs
Supper	12 oz glass of water, Pork tenderloin, spinach, olives, scallions, fresh lettuce salad, vinegar and oil 12 oz glass of water, tea 12 oz glass of water, tea	Half cup spinach—3.25 grams carbs 4 black olives—1 grams carbs 2 tablespoons scallions—1 gram carb 1 cup of salad greens—2 grams carbs
Day Eighteen	Before bed 12 oz glass of water, if you wake up in the night, drink 12 oz glass of water	Total carbohydrates = less than 30 grams carbs

Day Nineteen	**Meat Eaters Menu** Anyone may Eat as much protein as you want! SUBSTITUTE any PROTEIN with a Protein	**Carbohydrate Grams** Just Limit your Carbohydrates to 30 grams per day!
breakfast	at wake up—12 oz. glass of water, steak and eggs, salt, one cup black coffee, or tea 12 oz glass of water, vitamins	zero carbs
Break	12 oz glass of water, celery	2 stalks celery—3.2 grams carbs
Lunch	12 oz glass of water, lamb chops, cucumbers, tomato, fresh green salad (vinegar and oil) one cup black coffee or tea 12 oz glass of water	Half cucumber—1.8 grams carbs 1 tomato—5.8 grams carbs, 1 cup of salad greens— 2 grams carbs
Break	12 oz glass of water, two hard boiled eggs	zero carbs
Supper	12 oz glass of water, Pork roast, wild rice, mushrooms, fresh green salad (vinegar and oil) 12 oz glass of water	Half cup wild rice— 11 grams carbs Half cup mushrooms— 1.6 gram carb 1 cup of salad greens— 2 grams carbs
Day Nineteen	Before bed 12 oz glass of water, if you wake up in the night, drink 12 oz glass of water	Total carbohydrates = less than 30 grams carbs

	Meat Eaters Menu Anyone may Eat as much protein as you want! SUBSTITUTE any PROTEIN with a Protein	Carbohydrate Grams Just Limit your Carbohydrates to 30 grams per day!
Day Twenty		
breakfast	at wake up—12 oz. glass of water, cottage cheese and eggs one cup black coffee, or tea, 12 oz glass of water, vitamins	half cup cottage cheese— 4 grams carbs
Break	12 oz glass of water, nuts	3 tablespoons of mixed nuts— 7 grams carbs
Lunch	12 oz glass of water, hamburger patty with mushrooms fresh green salad with vinegar and oil, one cup black coffee or tea 12 oz glass of water	Half cup mushrooms— 1.6 grams carbs 1 cup of salad greens— 2 grams carbs
Break	12 oz glass of water, celery and cream cheese	2 stalks celery—3.2 grams carbs 2 tablespoons cream cheese— 1 grams carbs
Supper	12 oz glass of water, Roast beef, broccoli or Brussels sprouts fresh let- tuce, with vinegar and oil 12 oz glass of water, tea	Half cup broccoli— 4.25 grams carbs Half cup Brussels sprouts— 5 grams carbs 1 cup of salad greens— 2 grams carbs
Day Twenty	Before bed 12 oz glass of water, if you wake up in the night, drink 12 oz glass of water	Total carbohydrates = less than 30 grams carbs

Day Twenty One	Meat Eaters Menu Anyone may Eat as much protein as you want! SUBSTITUTE any PROTEIN with a Protein	Carbohydrate Grams Just Limit your Carbohydrates to 30 grams per day!
breakfast	at wake up—12 oz. glass of water, Sausage, and eggs salt, one cup black coffee, or tea, 12 oz glass of water, vitamins	half cup cottage cheese— 4 grams carbs
Break	12 oz glass of water, cheese	5 oz cheese—3 grams carbs
Lunch	12 oz glass of water, fish or seafood, cole slaw, fresh salad greens, black olives, tomato (vinegar and oil) one cup black coffee or tea 12 oz glass of water	Half cup cole slaw— 4.25 grams carbs 4 black olives—1 grams carbs 1 cup of salad greens— 2 grams carbs
Break	12 oz glass of water, cheese	5 oz cheese—3 grams carbs
Supper	12 oz glass of water, Beef tenderloin (or other lean cut) asparagus spears with cheese fresh green salad (vinegar and oil) 12 oz glass of water, tea	8 asparagus spears— 4.4 grams carbs grams carbs 5 oz cheese—5 grams carbs 1 cup of salad greens— 2 grams carbs
Day Twenty One	Before bed 12 oz glass of water, if you wake up in the night, drink 12 oz glass of water	Total carbohydrates = less than 30 grams carbs

Day Twenty Two	**Meat Eaters Menu** Anyone may Eat as much protein as you want! SUBSTITUTE any PROTEIN with a Protein	**Carbohydrate Grams** Just Limit your Carbohydrates to 30 grams per day!
breakfast	at wake up—12 oz. glass of water, Bacon [not sugar cured] and eggs [little salt/pepper] one cup black coffee, or tea, 12 oz glass of water, vitamins	zero carbohydrates
Break	12 oz glass of water, two hard boiled eggs	Break zero carbohydrates
Lunch	12 oz glass of water, shish kebab green salad (vinegar and oil) one cup black coffee or tea 12 oz glass of water	shish kabob vegetables— 20 grams carbs estimated 1 cup of salad greens— 2 grams carbs
Break	12 oz glass of water, tofu	zero carbohydrates
Supper	12 oz glass of water, corned beef and cabbage, fresh green salad (vinegar and oil) 12 oz glass of water, tea	1 cup cabbage— 6.2 grams carbs grams carbs 1 cup of salad greens— 2 grams carbs
Day Twenty Two	Before bed 12 oz glass of water, if you wake up in the night, drink 12 oz glass of water	Total carbohydrates = less than 30 grams carbs

Day Twenty Three	Meat Eaters Menu Anyone may Eat as much protein as you want! SUBSTITUTE any PROTEIN with a Protein	Carbohydrate Grams Just Limit your Carbohydrates to 30 grams per day!
breakfast	at wake up—12 oz. glass of water, cheese omelet with celery and peppers one cup black coffee, or tea, 12 oz glass of water, vitamins	3 oz cheese—1.8 grams carbs 1 stalk of celery— 1.6 grams carbs Quarter cup green peppers— 1.8 grams carbs
Break	12 oz glass of water, nuts	3 tablespoons mixed nuts— 7 grams carbs
Lunch	12 oz glass of water, steak and eggs, salt, fresh green salad (vinegar and oil) one cup black coffee or tea 12 oz glass of water	1 cup of salad greens— 2 grams carbs
Break	12 oz glass of water, nuts	3 tablespoons mixed nuts— 7 grams carbs
Supper	12 oz glass of water, fish with cucumbers, mushrooms, peppers fresh green salad (vinegar and oil) 12 oz glass of water, tea	Half cucumber—1.8 grams carbs Half cup mushrooms— 1.6 grams carbs Half pepper—3.6 grams carbs 1 cup of salad greens— 2 grams carbs
Day Twenty Three	Before bed 12 oz glass of water, if you wake up in the night, drink 12 oz glass of water,	Total carbohydrates = less than 30 grams carbs

	Meat Eaters Menu Anyone may Eat as much protein as you want! SUBSTITUTE any PROTEIN with a Protein	Carbohydrate Grams Just Limit your Carbohydrates to 30 grams per day!
Day Twenty Four		
breakfast	at wake up—12 oz. glass of water, Bacon [not sugar cured] and eggs, salt, one cup black coffee, or tea, 12 oz glass of water, vitamins	zero carbs
Break	12 oz glass of water, cheese	2 oz cheese—1.2 grams carbs
Lunch	12 oz glass of water, pork chops, cottage cheese, fresh green salad (vinegar and oil) one cup black coffee or tea 12 oz glass of water,	1 cup cottage cheese—8 grams carbs 1 cup of salad greens—2 grams carbs
Break	12 oz glass of water, nuts	3 tablespoons mixed nuts—7 grams carbs
Supper	12 oz glass of water, baked ham, collard greens, cabbage coleslaw or fresh green salad (vinegar and oil) 12 oz glass of water, tea	Half cup collard greens—.4.9 grams carbs Half cup cole slaw—4.25 grams carbs 1 cup of salad greens—2 grams carbs
Day Twenty Four	Before bed 12 oz glass of water, if you wake up in the night, drink 12 oz glass of water,	Total carbohydrates = less than 30 grams carbs

Day Twenty Five	Meat Eaters Menu Anyone may Eat as much protein as you want! SUBSTITUTE any PROTEIN with a Protein	Carbohydrate Grams Just Limit your Carbohydrates to 30 grams per day!
breakfast	at wake up—12 oz. glass of water, eggs and sausage, salt, one cup black coffee, or tea, 12 oz glass of water, vitamins	zero carbs
Break	12 oz glass of water, celery with cream cheese and nuts	3 stalks celery—4.8 grams carbs 3 tablespoons cream cheese—1.5 grams carbs One and half tablespoons of mixed nuts—3.5 grams carbs
Lunch	12 oz glass of water, steak with eggs fresh green salad (vinegar and oil) one cup black coffee or tea 12 oz glass of water,	1 cup of salad greens— 2 grams carbs
Break	12 oz glass of water, nuts	3 tablespoons mixed nuts— 7 grams carbs
Supper	12 oz glass of water, prime roast beef with mushrooms and snap green, fresh green salad (vinegar and oil) 12 oz glass of water, tea	Half cup snap greens— 3.4 grams carbs Half cup mushrooms— 1.6 grams carbs 1 cup of salad greens— 2 grams carbs
Day Twenty Five	Before bed 12 oz glass of water, if you wake up in the night, drink 12 oz glass of water	Total carbohydrates = less than 30 grams carbs

	Meat Eaters Menu	Carbohydrate Grams
Day Twenty Six	Anyone may Eat as much protein as you want! SUBSTITUTE any PROTEIN with a Protein	Just Limit your Carbohydrates to 30 grams per day!
breakfast	at wake up—12 oz. glass of water, cheese omelet, one cup black coffee, or tea, 12 oz glass of water, vitamins	3 Oz cheese—1.8 grams carbs
Break	12-oz glass of water, nuts with celery	3 stalks celery—4.8 grams carbs One and half tablespoons of mixed nuts—3.5 grams carbs
Lunch	12 oz glass of water, chicken, Cole slaw (no sugar in dressing) fresh green salad (vinegar and oil) one cup black coffee or tea 12 oz glass of water	Half cup cole slaw— 4.25 grams carbs 1 cup of salad greens— 2 grams carbs
Break	12 oz glass of water, nuts	2 tablespoons mixed nuts— 4.6 grams carbs
Supper	12 oz glass of water, Sirloin steak, mushrooms, asparagus spears & butter green salad (vinegar and oil) 12 oz glass of water	8 asparagus spears— 4.4 grams carbs Half cup mushrooms— 1.6 grams carbs 1 cup of salad greens— 2 grams carbs
Day Twenty Six	Before bed 12 oz glass of water, if you wake up in the night, drink 12 oz glass of water	Total carbohydrates = less than 30 grams carbs

Day Twenty Seven	Meat Eaters Menu Anyone may Eat as much protein as you want! SUBSTITUTE any PROTEIN with a Protein	Carbohydrate Grams Just Limit your Carbohydrates to 30 grams per day!
breakfast	at wake up—12 oz. glass of water, Canadian bacon [not sugar cured] & eggs one cup black coffee, or tea, 12 oz glass of water, vitamins	zero carbs
Break	12 oz glass of water, cheese and nuts	3 Oz cheese—1.8 grams carbs One and half tablespoons of mixed nuts—3.5 grams carbs
Lunch	12 oz glass of water, chicken, Cole slaw (no sugar in dressing) fresh green salad (vinegar and oil) one cup black coffee or tea 12 oz glass of water	Half cup cole slaw—4.25 grams carbs 1 cup of salad greens—2 grams carbs
Break	12 oz glass of water, celery with cream cheese and nuts	3 stalks celery—4.8 grams carbs 3 tablespoons cream cheese—1.5 grams carbs One and half tablespoons of mixed nuts—3.5 grams carbs
Supper	12 oz glass of water, chef salad with meat (vinegar and oil) 12 oz glass of water, tea	chef salad approximately 7 grams carbs
Day Twenty Seven	Before bed 12 oz glass of water, if you wake up in the night, drink 12 oz glass of water	Total carbohydrates = less than 30 grams carbs

Day Twenty Eight	Meat Eaters Menu Anyone may Eat as much protein as you want! SUBSTITUTE any PROTEIN with a Protein	Carbohydrate Grams Just Limit your Carbohydrates to 30 grams per day!
breakfast	at wake up—12 oz. glass of water, bacon [not sugar cured] and eggs, salt, one cup black coffee, or tea, 12 oz glass of water, vitamins	zero carbs
Break	12 oz glass of water, two hard boiled eggs	zero carbs
Lunch	12 oz glass of water, salmon with broccoli, fresh green salad (vinegar and oil) one cup black coffee or tea 12 oz glass of water	1 cup cole broccoli—7 grams carbs 1 cup of salad greens—2 grams carbs
Break	12 oz glass of water, celery with cream cheese and nuts	3 stalks celery—4.8 grams carbs 3 tablespoons cream cheese—1.5 grams carbs One and half tablespoons of mixed nuts—3.5 grams carbs
Supper	12 oz glass of water, Pork loin with asparagus with melted cheese, fresh green salad (vinegar and oil) 12 oz glass of water, tea	8 spears asparagus—4.4 grams carbs 3 oz cheese—1.8 grams carbs 1 cup of salad greens—2 grams carbs
Day Twenty Eight	Before bed 12 oz glass of water, if you wake up in the night, drink 12 oz glass of water	Total carbohydrates = less than 30 grams carbs

	Meat Eaters Menu Anyone may Eat as much protein as you want! SUBSTITUTE any PROTEIN with a Protein	Carbohydrate Grams Just Limit your Carbohydrates to 30 grams per day!
Day Twenty Nine		
breakfast	at wake up—12 oz. glass of water, tofu or eggs and cottage cheese one cup black coffee or tea, 12 oz glass of water, vitamins	zero carbs
Break	12 oz glass of water, two hard boiled eggs	zero carbs
Lunch	12 oz glass of water, fish and peppers, broccoli, fresh green salad (vinegar and oil), one cup black coffee or tea 12 oz glass of water	1 cup broccoli—7 grams carbs Half cup peppers—3.6 grams carbs 1 cup of salad greens—2 grams carbs
Break	12 oz glass of water, celery with cream cheese and nuts	3 stalks celery—4.8 grams carbs 3 tablespoons cream cheese—1.5 grams carbs One and half tablespoons of mixed nuts—3.5 grams carbs
Supper	12 oz glass of water, steak and asparagus, fresh green salad (vinegar and oil) 12 oz glass of water, tea	8 spears asparagus—4.4 grams carbs 1 cup of salad greens—2 grams carbs
Day Twenty Nine	Before bed 12 oz glass of water, if you wake up in the night, drink 12 oz glass of water	Total carbohydrates = less than 30 grams carbs

Day Thirty	Meat Eaters Menu Anyone may Eat as much protein as you want! SUBSTITUTE any PROTEIN with a Protein	Carbohydrate Grams Just Limit your Carbohydrates to 30 grams per day!
breakfast	at wake up—12 oz. glass of water, steak and eggs, salt, one cup black coffee, or tea, 12 oz glass of water, vitamin	zero carbs
Break	12 oz glass of water, two hard boiled eggs	zero carbs
Lunch	12 oz glass of water, lamb chops, cucumbers, tomato, mushrooms fresh green salad (vinegar and oil) one cup black coffee or tea 12 oz glass of water	Half cup cucumbers—1.8 grams carbs Half cup mushrooms—1.5 grams carbs Half tomato—2.9 grams carbs 1 cup of salad greens—2 grams carbs
Break	12 oz glass of water, celery with cream cheese	2 stalks celery—3.2 grams carbs 2 tablespoons cream cheese—1 grams carbs
Supper	12 oz glass of water, Pork roast, wild rice, mushrooms fresh green salad (vinegar and oil) 12 oz glass of water, tea	Third cup wild rice—14 grams carbs Half cup mushrooms—1.5 grams carbs 1 cup of salad greens—2 grams carbs
Day Thirty	Before bed 12 oz glass of water, if you wake up in the night, drink 12 oz glass of water	Total carbohydrates = less than 30 grams carbs

Vegetarians

Vegetarians have been eating a high carbohydrate diet, so this will be difficult but not impossible. The advantage you have as a vegetarian is you have demonstrated your will power by being a vegetarian. The key is to up your protein intake by eating vegetables high in protein, substituting all simple carbohydrates for non-starchy complex carbohydrates, avoiding fruits high in sugar and most important, any type SUGAR! What I have found is vegetarians eat a lot of fruit and sugar! Vegetarians with will power can modify *The Diet* by eating more protein and reducing carbohydrates to 30 grams a day, a daunting task, but not impossible.

Why would you even try this diet since you have already chosen to be a vegetarian? The only possible reason is either you want to lose weight or you want to feel healthier. I have found that vegetarians are usually not obese so I doubt if your motive is to lose weight. But if you have been eating tons of sugar and starches you may have a weight problem and this vegetarian diet will prove to you that you can lose weight! *The Diet* will prove also that you can feel healthier if you up your protein. Once you have proven this to yourself, you can then decide what to do about your protein deficiency. The *30-Day Vegetarian Diet Plan* is simply to prove to yourself that you need more protein. After the thirty days you can return to your previous vegetarian diet and see the difference. You will decide from this experiment whether or not you need more protein in your diet by the way you feel or if you lose some weight or both. The only way to know is try it. It is only thirty days of your life.

If you are an orthodox vegetarian [a vegan who avoids all products of animal origin, including milk and eggs] the highest source of protein in the vegetable world is soy, and eating soy products for a month isn't a feast, but also isn't a famine. Consider it a soy fast! There are a number of soy products on the market now that substitute meat and cheese which you no doubt are aware of. If you know of another source of vegetable in higher protein power than soy let me know. Depending on your orthodox vegetarian beliefs, you may eat eggs and cheese for thirty days along with the soy products. However, if you are a liberal vegetarian (an ovo-lacto vegetarian allowing eggs or dairy or a vegetarian allowing fowl, fish or shellfish) this makes the task easier to reduce your carbohydrates to 30 grams a day and have more variety in protein. If you are an orthodox vegetarian [vegan], is it possible to change your beliefs for just thirty days and be a liberal vegetarian allowing fowl, fish, or shellfish for the sake of losing weight or feeling better? It is just for thirty days! If this is not possible set your mind on a soy fast for thirty days! If you can eat eggs, consider an egg fast for thirty days! Orthodox vegetarians should either substitute soy or eggs for the PROTEINS suggested in the thirty-day diet plan or simply add them to the menu. You can eat as many eggs or as much protein powder as you want as long as the **protein powder has zero carbohydrates**. After the thirty days, you can eat whatever you want. Here are some suggestions on protein powder:

Trader Joe's Soy Protein Powder uses a "soy isolate," the chemistry used to isolate the soy that may have health ramifications for some, so I have included here three organic alternatives:

Iso-Rich Soy has 0 grams of sugar per 2 rounded tablespoons (28 g) of powder with water
Fermented Soy Essence™ has 2 grams of sugar per 2 rounded tablespoons (28 g) with water
Iso-Rich Soy Greens™ has 0 grams of sugar has per 2 tablespoons (31 g) of powder with water

The above three products are available at the following url:

http://www.jarrow.com

Remember to use just water or any liquid with zero carbohydrates such as cream with your protein powder. NO JUICE! Juice has too many carbohydrates.

Liberal vegetarians may substitute the vegetables suggested in the thirty-day diet plan with soy products that contain no sugar such as tofu, protein powder without any carbohydrates or sugar substitutes, fowl, fish, or shellfish, if allowed. So liberal vegetarians have more variety during the thirty days. For carbohydrates you may use dairy products (without fruit or sugar) and the vegetables mentioned at the end of this chapter. Avoid fruits and vegetables that are high in sugar content such as, potatoes (any color), white rice, corn, popcorn, cornbread, cornmeal, carrots, beets, white flour, and pasta which are all high in carbohydrates. Eat whole grains without sugar, honey, or any other sweetener during this thirty-day diet plan [ABSOLUTELY NO WHITE FLOUR] and no sugar substitutes. But remember no matter what carbohydrates you eat, the TOTAL NUMBER OF GRAMS PER DAY SHOULD BE LESS THAN 30 GRAMS! **You have the same carbohydrate limit as meat eaters**. For example, if you choose to eat one slice of whole wheat bread, which contains 11 grams of carbohydrate, you only have 19 grams left of carbohydrate to eat for the whole day! One cup of milk contains 11 grams of carbs. I know this is not easy, but vegetarians who wish to control their weight and feel healthy with their diet must have will power. If you can, avoid grains entirely for thirty days.

Avoid raisins, bananas, all fruits high in carbohydrates, fruit juices, parsnips, honey, carrots, corn/cornflakes, corn products, millet, beets, white rice, pasta, plain crackers, all types of white flour, any potatoes (any color), oatmeal or WHITE breads JUST FOR THIRTY DAYS. It will be extremely difficult to only eat 30 grams of carbohydrates a day, but it can be done by an orthodox vegetarian with will power. For example, two scoops (28 grams) of Trader Joe's Soy Protein Powder have 1 gram of fat and 23 grams of protein with ZERO carbohydrates. That gives you an idea of how to do it. Depending on what type of vegetarian you are, substitute the meats in *The Diet* with eggs, cheese, fish, fowl, shellfish, or soy products. An excellent source to count carbohydrate grams is found in the chapter on *Reading the Nutrition Label.*

Vegans usually are aware of the lack of vitamin B12 in the their diet. B12 is generally assumed to be found only in animal products. B12 is difficult to obtain from plants but does occur in some fermented plant foods, such as tempeh, miso, etc. A B12 supplement can help assure adequate amounts in the vegan diet. B12 occurs as a molecule with an atom of cobalt at its center but does not technically come from animals or plants since microorganisms such as bacteria and algae make it. These are found in and on the foods we eat. The bacteria in the livestock's digestive system spread the B12 vitamin throughout the flesh and milk. If you are a vegetarian who eats eggs and dairy products you will get B12 in your diet. If you are a vegan, you should think about B12 supplements. More information on B12 can be found at this url >

http://www.earthsave.bc.ca/materials/articles/health/b12.html

Soy is the only known plant with all nine essential amino acids and is an excellent source of protein for vegans (see the chapters, Protein and Protein Synthesis). For thirty days vegetarians should eat a high protein diet to lose weight or feel healthier. If after thirty days you notice a difference you may want to seriously consider whether your current diet is protein deficient and decide what to do about it. The 30-Day Diet Plan for Vegetarians is for vegans. If you can add protein such as fish, fowl, eggs, or dairy then you have additional sources in whatever amounts you want since these sources of protein rarely have any carbohydrate.

Vegetarians may substitute any of the following:

Fish or Shell Fish (if allowed)
Fowl—i.e., chicken or Turkey (if allowed)
Eggs
Soy Products (soy milk, cereals with no sugar, soy burgers, soy links, etc., note any carbohydrate in the product and add into the 30 grams a day limit)
Soy Protein Powder with ZERO carbohydrates or sugar/sugar substitutes
Protein Powder (egg or other source acceptable to you) with no sugar/sugar substitutes that contains zero carbohydrates on the Nutrition Facts Label
Tofu, Tempeh, Miso
Nonstarchy vegetables low in carbohydrates
asparagus, bamboo shoots, bean sprouts, bok choy, broccoli, cabbage, chinese cabbage, cauliflower, celery, collards, cucumber, dandelion greens, egg plant, endive, escarole, garlic, green pepper, kale, lettuce, mushrooms, mustard greens, okra, onions, parsley, peppers, tomatoes, radishes, snow peas, sauerkraut, spinach, summer squash, swis chard, tomatoes, turnip greens, turnips, scallions
Fruit lowest in carbohydrates
acerola, apricots, avocados, kumquat, lemon, lime, grapefruits, plums, prune
Dairy Products without sugar
butter, cream, cheese, whole milk cottage cheese, cream cheese, milk, ricotta, sour cream, plain whole milk yogurt
Legumes
black-eyed peas, canellini beans, chickpeas, green snap beans, yellow snap beans, kidney beans, lentils, lima beans, peanuts, and soybeans
NUTS & Seeds

The following Vegetarian 30 Day Diet Plan is designed for vegans, those vegetarians who will not eat any animal food whether dairy, fish, seafood, fowl, meat or eggs. If you are a more liberal vegetarian add fish, fowl, seafood, dairy or eggs to the suggested menu you may eat as much as you want of these items since there is usually no carbohydrate in these sources of protein. By now you must hate my repetition, but for some reason I still get frequently asked questions about this. Weird isn't it?

You may substitute any protein with a protein. I have suggested some name brand products that were available on the East Coast and you may have to substitute an item with what products you have available in your area. These name brand products are all vegan. The main idea is to give you a menu suggestion for thirty days and you can freely substitute what you want or have available. You may also substitute a carbohydrate with another carbohydrate as long as you stay with the 30 grams a day limit for thirty days. At the end of the thirty days you may of course, as the diet authority, eat whatever you want. Vegetarians usually have more will power than omnivores but sometimes have difficulty giving up sweets and fruits. Can you do it? It is only for thirty days.

	Vegetarian Menu Eat as much protein as you want! SUBSTITUTE any PROTEIN with a Protein Liberal Vegetarians may add dairy products such as cheese, cream, eggs, or any seafood, fish, or fowl and eat as much as you want!	Carbohydrate Grams Just Limit your Carbohydrates To 30 Grams per day!
Day One		
breakfast	at wake up—12 oz. glass of water, Tofu, salt, one cup black coffee or tea, 12 oz glass of water, vitamins	4 inch cube tofu— 5.8 grams carbs
Break	12 oz glass of water, celery	2 stalks celery—3.2 grams carbs
Lunch	12 oz glass of water, 1/2 avocado, fresh salad greens, black olives, tomato (vinegar and oil), protein pow- der, one cup black coffee or tea, 12 oz glass of water	half California avocado— 6.5 grams carbs, 4 black olives—1 gram carb, 1 cup of salad greens— 2 grams carbs Half tomato—3 grams carbs
Break	12 oz glass of water, celery	2 stalks celery—3.2 grams carbs
Supper	12 oz glass of water, protein powder, asparagus spears, fresh green salad, (vinegar and oil) tea, 12 oz. glass of water	4 fresh asparagus spears— 2.2 grams carbs 1 cup of salad—2 grams carbs
Day One	Before bed 12 oz glass of water, if you wake up in the night, drink 12 oz glass of water	Total carbohydrates = Less than 30 grams carbs

Day Two	Vegetarian Menu Eat as much protein as you want! SUBSTITUTE any PROTEIN with a Protein Liberal Vegetarians may add dairy products such as cheese, cream, eggs, or any seafood, fish, or fowl and eat as much as you want!	Carbohydrate Grams Just Limit your Carbohydrates to 30 grams per day!
breakfast	at wake up—12 oz. glass of water, protein powder, one cup black coffee or tea, 12 oz glass of water, vitamins	Zero carbs
Break	12 oz glass of water, cauliflower, mixed nuts	Half cup cauliflower—2.2 grams carbs On and half tablespoons mixed nuts—3.5 grams carbs
Lunch	12 oz glass of water, fresh green salad (vinegar and oil) with tomato, toffutti, one cup black coffee or tea, 12 oz glass of water	Toffutti—2 slices of soy mozzarella slices—2 grams carbs 1 cup of salad greens—2 grams carbs Whole tomato—6 grams carbs
Break	12 oz glass of water, Sunergia Soyfoods, More than Tofu	Sunergia Soyfoods, More than Tofu Indian Masala—2 oz—3 grams carbs
Supper	12 oz glass of water, tofu, cabbage cole slaw or fresh green salad (vinegar and oil) 12 oz glass of water, tea	4 inch cube tofu—5.8 grams carbs, Half cup cole slaw w/dressing—.2.5 grams carbs 1 cup of salad greens—2 grams carbs
Day Two	Before bed 12 oz glass of water, if you wake up in the night, drink 12 oz glass of water	Total carbohydrates = Less than 30 grams carbs

	Vegetarian Menu Eat as much protein as you want! SUBSTITUTE any PROTEIN with a Protein Liberal Vegetarians may add dairy products such as cheese, cream, eggs, or any seafood, fish, or fowl and eat as much as you want!	**Carbohydrate Grams** Just Limit your Carbohydrates to 30 grams per day!
Day Three		
breakfast	at wake up—12 oz. glass of water, protein powder, grapefruit, one cup black coffee or tea 12 oz glass of water, vitamins	Half grapefruit—3 in dia.—10.3 grams carbs
break	12 oz glass of water, nuts with celery	1 tablespoon mixed nuts— 2 grams carbs 2 stalks celery—3 grams carbs
Lunch	12 oz glass of water, Cole slaw (no sugar in dressing) or fresh green salad (vinegar and oil), Soya Kaas, one cup black coffee or tea 12 oz glass of water	Half cup cole slaw w/dressing— 2 Grams carbs Soya Kaas Mozzarella Style Natural Cheese Alternative—2 oz less than 2 grams carbs 1 cup of salad greens— 2 grams carbs
Break	12 oz glass of water, celery, protein powder	2 stalks celery—3 grams carbs
Supper	12 oz glass of water, protein powder, cabbage, fresh green salad (vinegar and oil) 12 oz glass of water, tea	Half cabbage—2.2 grams carbs 1 cup of salad greens— 2 grams carbs
Day Three	Before bed 12 oz glass of water, if you wake up in the night, drink 12 oz glass of water	Total carbohydrates = Less than 30 grams carbs

Day Four	Vegetarian Menu Eat as much protein as you want! SUBSTITUTE any PROTEIN with a Protein Liberal Vegetarians may add dairy products such as cheese, cream, eggs, or any seafood, fish, or fowl and eat as much as you want!	Carbohydrate Grams Just Limit your Carbohydrates to 30 grams per day!
breakfast	at wake up—12 oz. glass of water, celery and peanut or almond butter, salt, one cup black coffee or tea, 12 oz glass of water, vitamins	2 teaspoons peanut butter or one quarter of ounce almond butter—6 grams carbs 3 stalks celery—4.8 grams carbs
Break	12 oz glass of water, fresh cabbage	1 cup raw cabbage—4.9 grams carbs
Lunch	12 oz glass of water, green salad (vinegar and oil) with green pepper, one cup black coffee or tea 12 oz glass of water	Half cup green pepper—3 grams carbs 1 cup of salad greens—2 grams carbs
Break	12 oz glass of water, protein powder	Zero carbs
Supper	12 oz glass of water, cooked cabbage, fresh green salad (vinegar and oil) 12 oz glass of water, tea	1 cup cooked cabbage—6 grams carbs 1 cup of salad greens—2 grams carbs
Day Four	Before bed 12 oz glass of water, if you wake up in the night, drink 12 oz glass of water	Total carbohydrates = Less than 30 grams carbs

	Vegetarian Menu Eat as much protein as you want! SUBSTITUTE any PROTEIN with a Protein Liberal Vegetarians may add dairy products such as cheese, cream, eggs, or any seafood, fish, or fowl and eat as much as you want!	Carbohydrate Grams Just Limit your Carbohydrates to 30 grams per day!
Day Five		
breakfast	at wake up—12 oz. glass of water, protein powder, one cup black coffee or tea, 12 oz glass of water, vitamins	Zero carbs
Break	12 oz glass of water, nuts, protein powder	1 tablespoon of Mixed nuts— 2.3 grams carbs
Lunch	12 oz glass of water, fresh green salad (vinegar and oil), tomato, Smart Dogs!, one cup black coffee or tea 12 oz glass of water	1 cup of salad greens— 2 grams carbs half tomato—3 grams carbs Smart Dogs! Meat Free soy Protein Links—2 links— 10 grams carbs
Break	12 oz glass of water, celery with mixed nuts, protein powder	2 stalks celery—3.2 grams carbs 1 tablespoon mixed nuts— 2.3 grams carbs
Supper	12 oz glass of water, salad (vinegar and oil), tomato, protein powder, 12 oz glass of water, tea	salad—2 grams carbs half tomato—3 grams carbs
Day Five	Before bed 12 oz glass of water, if you wake up in the night, drink 12 oz glass of water	Total carbohydrates = around 30 grams carbs

Day Six	Vegetarian Menu Eat as much protein as you want! SUBSTITUTE any PROTEIN with a Protein Liberal Vegetarians may add dairy products such as cheese, cream, eggs, or any seafood, fish, or fowl and eat as much as you want!	Carbohydrate Grams Just Limit your Carbohydrates to 30 grams per day!
breakfast	at wake up—12 oz. glass of water, protein powder, one cup black coffee or tea, 12 oz glass of water, vitamins	Zero carbs
Break	12 oz glass of water, celery and nuts	2 tablespoons of Mixed nuts—4.6 grams carbs 2 stalks celery—3.2 grams carbs
Lunch	12 oz glass of water, cooked spinach, fresh green salad (vinegar and oil) Veggy Singles, one cup black coffee or tea 12 oz glass of water	One cup cooked spinach—6.5 grams carbs 1 cup of salad greens—2 grams carbs Veggy singles (Pepper Jack, cheddar or mazzarella)—30 grams—1 gram carbs
Break	12 oz glass of water, protein powder and nuts	2 tablespoons of Mixed nuts—4.6 grams carbs
Supper	12 oz glass of water, fresh green salad (vinegar and oil) with eggplant 12 oz glass of water	Half cup eggplant—4.1 grams carbs 1 cup of salad greens—2 grams carbs
Day Six	Before bed 12 oz glass of water, if you wake up in the night, drink 12 oz glass of water	Total carbohydrates = less than 30 grams carbs

	Vegetarian Menu Eat as much protein as you want! SUBSTITUTE any PROTEIN with a Protein Liberal Vegetarians may add dairy products such as cheese, cream, eggs, or any seafood, fish, or fowl and eat as much as you want!	Carbohydrate Grams Just Limit your Carbohydrates to 30 grams per day!
Day Seven		
breakfast	at wake up—12 oz. glass of water, protein powder, one cup black coffee or tea, 12 oz glass of water, vitamins	Zero carbs
Break	12 oz glass of water, protein powder	zero carbs
Lunch	12 oz glass of water, peppers, broccoli, fresh green salad (vinegar and oil) with fresh turnip greens, tomato, one cup black coffee or tea 12 oz glass of water	Half cup diced peppers— 3 grams carbs Half cup broccoli— 3.5 grams carbs Half cup turnip greens— 2.6 grams carbs 1 cup of salad greens— 2 grams carbs whole tomato—5.8 grams carbs
Break	12 oz glass of water, celery and nuts, protein powder	2 stalks celery—3.2 grams carbs 1 tablespoon mixed nuts— 2.9 grams carbs
Supper	12 oz glass of water, asparagus, fresh green salad (vinegar and oil), Smart Deli, 12 oz glass of water	4 asparagus spears— 2.2 grams carbs 1 cup of salad greens— 2 grams carbs Smart Deli Old World bologna Style Meatless Slices—3 slices—2 grams carbs
Day Seven	Before bed 12 oz glass of water, if you wake up in the night, drink 12 oz glass of water	Total carbohydrates = less than 30 grams carbs

Day Eight	**Vegetarian Menu** Eat as much protein as you want! SUBSTITUTE any PROTEIN with a Protein Liberal Vegetarians may add dairy products such as cheese, cream, eggs, or any seafood, fish, or fowl and eat as much as you want!	**Carbohydrate Grams** Just Limit your Carbohydrates to 30 grams per day!
breakfast	at wake up—12 oz. glass of water, Gimme Lean!, scrambled tofu, one cup black coffee or tea 12 oz glass of water, vitamins	Gimme Lean! Meatless Sausage Style—2 oz—4 grams carbs 2 inch cube tofu— 2.9 grams carbs
Break	12 oz glass of water, and nuts, protein powder	One and half tablespoons of mixed nuts—3.5 grams carbs
Lunch	12 oz glass of water, fresh green salad (vinegar and oil), protein powder, one cup black coffee or tea 12 oz glass of water	1 cup of salad greens— 2 grams carbs
Break	12 oz glass of water, celery with nuts	2 stalks celery—3.2 grams carbs One and half tablespoons of mixed nuts—3.5 grams carbs
Supper	12 oz glass of water, cucumbers, mushrooms, peppers fresh green salad (vinegar and oil), protein powder, 12 oz glass of water	Half cucumber—1.8 grams carbs Half cup mushrooms— 2.6 grams carbs Half cup green pepper— 3.6 grams carbs 1 cup of salad greens— 2 grams carbs
Day Eight	Before bed 12 oz glass of water, if you wake up in the night, drink 12 oz glass of water	Total carbohydrates = around 30 grams carbs

	Vegetarian Menu Eat as much protein as you want! SUBSTITUTE any PROTEIN with a Protein	Carbohydrate Grams Just Limit your Carbohydrates to 30 grams per day!
Day Nine	Liberal Vegetarians may add dairy products such as cheese, cream, eggs, or any seafood, fish, or fowl and eat as much as you want!	
breakfast	at wake up—12 oz. glass of water, Yves Veggie Cuisine, scrambled tofu, one cup black coffee or tea, 12 oz glass of water, vitamins	Yves Veggie Cuisine the Good Deli Veggie Ham Slices—2 slices—3 grams carbs 2 inch cube tofu— 2.9 grams carbs
Break	12 oz glass of water, nuts, protein powder	One and half tablespoons of mixed nuts—3.5 grams carbs
Lunch	12 oz glass of water, green peppers fresh green salad (vinegar and oil) protein powder, one cup black coffee or tea 12 oz glass of water	One pepper—7.2 grams carbs 1 cup of salad greens— 2 grams carbs
Break	12 oz glass of water, protein powder	zero carbs
Supper	12 oz glass of water, salad with whole tomato, (vinegar and oil) 12 oz glass of water, tea	salad—2 grams carbs whole tomato—5.8 grams carbs
Day Nine	Before bed 12 oz glass of water, if you wake up in the night, drink 12 oz glass of water	Total carbohydrates = less than 30 grams carbs

Day Ten	**Vegetarian Menu** Eat as much protein as you want! SUBSTITUTE any PROTEIN with a Protein Liberal Vegetarians may add dairy products such as cheese, cream, eggs, or any seafood, fish, or fowl and eat as much as you want!	**Carbohydrate Grams** Just Limit your Carbohydrates to 30 grams per day!
breakfast	at wake up—12 oz. glass of water, protein powder, coffee or tea, 12 oz glass of water, vitamins	zero carbs
Break	12 oz glass of water, nuts, protein powder	One and half tablespoons of mixed nuts—3.5 grams carbs
Lunch	12 oz glass of water, tofu, Miso Master Organic Red Miso, fresh green salad (vinegar and oil) one cup black coffee or tea 12 oz glass of water	2 inch cube tofu— 2.9 grams carbs Miso Master Organic Red Miso (Traditional soy Paste or Barley Miso)—2 tsp—2 grams carbs 1 cup of salad greens— 2 grams carbs
Break	12 oz glass of water, celery and nuts	2 stalks celery—3.2 grams carbs One and half tablespoons of mixed nuts—3.5 grams carbs
Supper	12 oz glass of water, mushrooms, zucchini, spinach fresh green salad (vinegar and oil), protein powder 12 oz glass of water	Half cup mushrooms— 1.5 grams carbs Half cup zucchini— 2.6 grams carbs 1 cup spinach—6.5 grams carbs
Day Ten	Before bed 12 oz glass of water, if you wake up in the night, drink 12 oz glass of water	Total carbohydrates = less than 30 grams carbs

	Vegetarian Menu Eat as much protein as you want! SUBSTITUTE any PROTEIN with a Protein Liberal Vegetarians may add dairy products such as cheese, cream, eggs, or any seafood, fish, or fowl and eat as much as you want!	Carbohydrate Grams Just Limit your Carbohydrates to 30 grams per day!
Day Eleven		
breakfast	at wake up—12 oz. glass of water, protein powder, one cup black coffee or tea, 12 oz glass of water, vitamins	Zero carbs
Break	12 oz glass of water, celery with Miso Master Organic Mellow White Soy Paste and nuts	3 stalks celery—4.8 grams carbs Miso Master Organic Mellow White Soy Paste—2 tsp—3 grams carbs One and half tablespoons of mixed nuts—3.5 grams carbs
Lunch	12 oz glass of water, green beans, fresh green salad (vinegar and oil), one cup black coffee or tea, 12 oz glass of water	Half cup green snap beans—3.4 grams/carb 1 cup of salad greens—2 grams carbs
Break	12 oz glass of water, protein powder	zero carbs
Supper	12 oz glass of water, spinach, fresh green salad (vinegar and oil), Smoke & Fire Soy with Sizzle Herb Smoked Tofu, 12 oz glass of water, tea	One cup cooked spinach—6.5 grams carbs 1 cup of salad greens—2 grams carbs Smoke & Fire Soy with Sizzle Herb Smoked Tofu—half cup—2 grams carbs
Day Eleven	Before bed 12 oz glass of water, if you wake up in the night, drink 12 oz glass of water	Total carbohydrates = less than 30 grams carbs

	Vegetarian Menu Eat as much protein as you want! SUBSTITUTE any PROTEIN with a Protein Liberal Vegetarians may add dairy products such as cheese, cream, eggs, or any seafood, fish, or fowl and eat as much as you want!	Carbohydrate Grams Just Limit your Carbohydrates to 30 grams per day!
Day Twelve		
breakfast	at wake up—12 oz. glass of water, Lightlife Fakin Bacon, scrambled tofu, one cup black coffee or tea, 12 oz glass of water, vitamins	Lightlife Fakin Bacon Marinated Smokey Tempeh Strips—3 slices —6 grams carbs 2 inch cube of tofu—2.9 carbs
Break	12 oz glass of water, celery with almond butter	2 stalks celery—3.2 grams carbs Quarter oz almond butter— 3.6 grams carbs
Lunch	12 oz glass of water, broccoli, fresh green salad (vinegar and oil), protein powder, one cup black coffee or tea 12 oz glass of water	Half cup broccoli— 3.5 grams/carb 1 cup of salad greens— 2 grams carbs
Break	12 oz glass of water, celery, protein powder	3 stalks celery—4.8 grams carbs
Supper	12 oz glass of water, asparagus, fresh green salad (vinegar and oil), protein powder 12 oz glass of water, tea	4 asparagus spears— 2.2 grams carbs 1 cup of salad greens— 2 grams carbs
Day Twelve	Before bed 12 oz glass of water, if you wake up in the night, drink 12 oz glass of water	Total carbohydrates = around 30 grams carbs

	Vegetarian Menu Eat as much protein as you want! SUBSTITUTE any PROTEIN with a Protein Liberal Vegetarians may add dairy products such as cheese, cream, eggs, or any seafood, fish, or fowl and eat as much as you want!	Carbohydrate Grams Just Limit your Carbohydrates to 30 grams per day!
Day Thirteen		
breakfast	at wake up—12 oz. glass of water, tempeh, one cup black coffee or tea, 12 oz glass of water, vitamins	2 oz. tempeh—7 grams carbs
Break	12 oz glass of water, celery and nuts	2 stalks celery—3.2 grams carbs One and half tablespoons of mixed nuts—3.5 grams carbs
Lunch	12 oz glass of water, eggplant, fresh green salad (vinegar and oil), protein powder, one cup black coffee or tea 12 oz glass of water	Half cup eggplant— 4.1 grams/carb 1 cup of salad greens— 2 grams carbs
Break	12 oz glass of water, nuts, protein powder	3 oz cheese—1.8 grams carbs One and half tablespoons of mixed nuts—3.5 grams carbs
Supper	12 oz glass of water, mushrooms, fresh green salad, protein powder, (vinegar and oil) 12 oz glass of water, tea	Half cup mushrooms— 2.5 gram/carb 1 cup of salad greens— 2 grams carbs
Day Thirteen	Before bed 12 oz glass of water, if you wake up in the night, drink 12 oz glass of water	Total carbohydrates = less than 30 grams carbs

Day Fourteen	**Vegetarian Menu** Eat as much protein as you want! SUBSTITUTE any PROTEIN with a Protein Liberal Vegetarians may add dairy products such as cheese, cream, eggs, or any seafood, fish, or fowl and eat as much as you want!	**Carbohydrate Grams** Just Limit your Carbohydrates to 30 grams per day!
breakfast	at wake up—12 oz. glass of water, scrambled tofu with celery and peppers. one cup black coffee or tea, 12 oz glass of water, vitamins	2 inch cube of tofu—2.9 grams carbs 1 stalk celery—1.6 grams carbs Half cup green pepper—3.6 grams carbs
Break	12 oz glass of water, nuts, protein powder	1 tablespoons of mixed nuts—2.3 grams carbs
Lunch	12 oz glass of water, eggplant with fresh green salad (vinegar and oil) one cup black coffee or tea 12 oz glass of water	Half cup eggplant—4.1 grams carbs 1 cup of salad greens—2 grams carbs
Break	12 oz glass of water, celery, South River Certified Organic Sweet Tasting Brown Rice Miso	2 stalks celery—2.4 grams carbs South River Certified Organic Sweet Tasting Brown Rice Miso—1 tsp—2 grams carbs
Supper	12 oz glass of water, Smoke and Fire Soy with Sizzle Lemon Garlic Smoked Tofu and mushrooms fresh green salad (vinegar and oil) 12 oz glass of water, tea	Smoke and Fire Soy with Sizzle Lemon Garlic Smoked Tofu—half cup—3 grams carbs Half cup mushrooms—2.5 gram carbs 1 cup of salad greens—2 grams carbs
Day Fourteen	Before bed 12 oz glass of water, if you wake up in the night, drink 12 oz glass of water	Total carbohydrates = around 30 grams carbs

	Vegetarian Menu Eat as much protein as you want! SUBSTITUTE any PROTEIN with a Protein	**Carbohydrate Grams**
Day Fifteen	Liberal Vegetarians may add cheese, cream, eggs, seafood, fish, or fowl as much as you want! Eat as much pro- tein as you want! SUBSTITUTE any PROTEIN with a Protein	Just Limit your Carbohydrates to 30 grams per day!
breakfast	at wake up—12 oz. glass of water, scrambled Smoke and Fire Soy with Sizzle Herb Smoked Tofu, one cup black coffee, or tea, 12 oz glass of water, vitamins	Smoke and Fire Soy with Sizzle Herb Smoked Tofu—half cup— 2 grams carbs
Break	12 oz glass of water, protein powder, nuts	1 tablespoons of mixed nuts— 2.3 grams carbs
Lunch	12 oz glass of water, spinach, fresh green salad with vinegar and oil, one cup black coffee or tea 12 oz glass of water	1 cup spinach—6.5 grams carb 1 cup of salad greens— 2 grams carbs
Break	12 oz glass of water, celery with South River Certified Organic Three- Year Barley Miso	3 stalks celery—4.8 grams carbs South River Certified Organic Three-Year Barley Miso— 3 tsp—3 grams carbs
Supper	12 oz glass of water, scallions, pep- pers, and fresh lettuce, grape toma- toes with vinegar and oil 12 oz glass of water, tea	2 tablespoons scallions— 2 grams carbs 1 cup of salad greens— 2 grams carbs 5 grape tomatoes— 3 grams carbs
Day Fifteen	Before bed 12 oz glass of water, if you wake up in the night, drink 12 oz glass of water	Total carbohydrates = less than 30 grams carbs

Day Sixteen	**Vegetarian Menu** Eat as much protein as you want! SUBSTITUTE any PROTEIN with a Protein Liberal Vegetarians may add dairy products such as cheese, cream, eggs, or any seafood, fish, or fowl and eat as much as you want!	**Carbohydrate Grams** Just Limit your Carbohydrates to 30 grams per day!
breakfast	at wake up—12 oz. glass of water, scrambled Smoke & Fire Soy with Sizzle Lemon Garlic Smoked Tofu, salt, one cup black coffee, or tea, 12 oz glass of water, vitamins	Smoke & Fire Soy with Sizzle Lemon Garlic Smoked Tofu—half cup—3 grams carbs
Break	12 oz glass of water, nuts, protein powder	2 tablespoons of mixed nuts—4.6 grams carbs
Lunch	12 oz glass of water, kale, protein powder, fresh green salad (vinegar and oil) one cup black coffee or tea 12 oz glass of water	half cup kale—3.4 grams carbs 1 cup of salad greens—2 grams carbs
Break	12 oz glass of water, protein powder	zero carbs
Supper	12 oz glass of water, protein powder, collard greens, fresh green salad with vinegar and oil, one cup black coffee or tea 12 oz glass of water	1 cup collards—9.8 grams carbs 1 cup of salad greens—2 grams carbs 5 grape tomatoes—3 grams carbs
Day Sixteen	Before bed 12 oz glass of water, if you wake up in the night, drink 12 oz glass of water	Total carbohydrates = less than 30 grams carbs

Day Seventeen	Vegetarian Menu Eat as much protein as you want! SUBSTITUTE any PROTEIN with a Protein Liberal Vegetarians may add dairy products such as cheese, cream, eggs, or any seafood, fish, or fowl and eat as much as you want!	Carbohydrate Grams Just Limit your Carbohydrates to 30 grams per day!
breakfast	at wake up—12 oz. glass of water, peanut butter with celery, cup black coffee, or tea, 12 oz glass of water, vitamins	2 Tablespoons of peanut butter—6 grams carbs 2 celery stalks—3.2 grams carbs
Break	12 oz glass of water, nuts, protein powder	2 tablespoons of mixed nuts—4.6 grams carbs
Lunch	12 oz glass of water, protein powder, green salad (vinegar and oil) with asparagus spears, melted cheddar Veggie Singles, one cup black coffee or tea 12 oz glass of water	4 asparagus spears—2.2 grams carbs 1 cup of salad greens—2 grams carbs Veggie Singles cheddar—30 grams portion—1 gram carbs
Break	12 oz glass of water, celery with peanut butter	2 stalks celery—3.2 grams carbs 2 tablespoons peanut butter—3.2 grams carbs
Supper	12 oz glass of water, protein powder, raw spinach, fresh green salad (vinegar and oil) 12 oz glass of water, tea	1 cup raw spinach—2.4 grams carbs 1 cup of salad greens—2 grams carbs
Day Seventeen	Before bed 12 oz glass of water, if you wake up in the night, drink 12 oz glass of water	Total carbohydrates = around 30 grams carbs

Day Eighteen	**Vegetarian Menu** Eat as much protein as you want! SUBSTITUTE any PROTEIN with a Protein Liberal Vegetarians may add dairy products such as cheese, cream, eggs, or any seafood, fish, or fowl and eat as much as you want!	**Carbohydrate Grams** Just Limit your Carbohydrates to 30 grams per day!
breakfast	at wake up—12 oz. glass of water, protein powder, salt, one cup black coffee, or tea, 2 oz glass of water, vitamins	Zero carbs
Break	12 oz glass of water, celery	3 celery stalks—4.8 grams carbs
Lunch	12 oz glass of water, turnip, fresh green salad with vinegar and oil, Smart Dogs! and sauerkraut, mustard, one cup black coffee or tea 12 oz glass of water	half cup turnip—.4.3 grams carbs 1 cup of salad greens—2 grams carbs Smart Dogs!—2 links—10 grams carbs
Break	12 oz glass of water, protein powder	zero carbs
Supper	12 oz glass of water, protein powder, spinach, olives, scallions, fresh lettuce salad, vinegar and oil 12 oz glass of water, tea 12 oz glass of water, tea	Half cup spinach—3.25 grams carbs 10 ripe olives—1.2 grams carbs 2 tablespoons scallions—1 gram/carb 1 cup of salad greens—2 grams carbs
Day Eighteen	Before bed 12 oz glass of water, if you wake up in the night, drink 12 oz glass of water	Total carbohydrates = less than 30 grams carbs

Day Nineteen	**Vegetarian Menu** Eat as much protein as you want! SUBSTITUTE any PROTEIN with a Protein Liberal Vegetarians may add dairy products such as cheese, cream, eggs, or any seafood, fish, or fowl and eat as much as you want!	**Carbohydrate Grams** Just Limit your Carbohydrates to 30 grams per day!
breakfast	at wake up—12 oz. glass of water, protein powder, one cup black coffee, or tea 12 oz glass of water, vitamins	zero carbs
Break	12 oz glass of water, celery	2 stalks celery—3.2 grams carbs
Lunch	12 oz glass of water, Smoke & Fire Soy with Sizzle BBQ Smoked, cucumbers, tomato, fresh green salad (vinegar and oil) one cup black coffee or tea 12 oz glass of water	Smoke & Fire Soy with Sizzle BBQ Smoked—half cup—3 grams carbs Half cucumber—1.8 grams carbs 1 tomato—5.8 grams carbs, 1 cup of salad greens—2 grams carbs
Break	12 oz glass of water, protein powder	zero carbs
Supper	12 oz glass of water, protein powder, wild rice, mushrooms, fresh green salad (vinegar and oil) 12 oz glass of water	Half cup wild rice—11 grams carbs Half cup mushrooms—1.6 gram carb 1 cup of salad greens—2 grams carbs
Day Nineteen	Before bed 12 oz glass of water, if you wake up in the night, drink 12 oz glass of water	Total carbohydrates = around 30 grams carbs

Day Twenty	**Vegetarian Menu** Eat as much protein as you want! SUBSTITUTE any PROTEIN with a Protein Liberal Vegetarians may add dairy products such as cheese, cream, eggs, or any seafood, fish, or fowl and eat as much as you want!	**Carbohydrate Grams** Just Limit your Carbohydrates to 30 grams per day!
breakfast	at wake up—12 oz. glass of water, protein powder, one cup black coffee or tea, 12 oz glass of water, vitamins	Zero carbs
Break	12 oz glass of water, nuts	2 tablespoons of mixed nuts—4.6 grams carbs
Lunch	12 oz glass of water, Light Life Foney Baloney, mushrooms with fresh green salad with vinegar and oil, one cup black coffee or tea 12 oz glass of water	Light Life Foney Baloney—3 slices—2 grams carbs Half cup mushrooms—1.6 grams carbs 1 cup of salad greens—2 grams carbs
Break	12 oz glass of water, celery and peanut butter	2 stalks celery—3.2 grams carbs 2 tablespoons cream cheese—6 grams carbs
Supper	12 oz glass of water, Roast beef, broccoli o, Brussels sprouts, fresh lettuce, with vinegar and oil 12 oz glass of water, tea	Half cup broccoli—3.5 grams carbs Half cup Brussels sprouts—4.5 gram/carb 1 cup of salad greens—2 grams carbs
Day Twenty	Before bed 12 oz glass of water, if you wake up in the night, drink 12 oz glass of water	Total carbohydrates = less than 30 grams carbs

Day Twenty One	Vegetarian Menu Eat as much protein as you want! SUBSTITUTE any PROTEIN with a Protein Liberal Vegetarians may add dairy products such as cheese, cream, eggs, or any seafood, fish, or fowl and eat as much as you want!	Carbohydrate Grams Just Limit your Carbohydrates to 30 grams per day!
breakfast	at wake up—12 oz. glass of water, scrambled tofu with Light Life Fakin Bacon Marinated Smokey Tempeh, one cup black coffee or tea, 12 oz glass of water, vitamins	2 inch cube tofu— 2.9 grams carbs Light Life Fakin Bacon Marinated Smokey Tempeh—3 slices— 6 grams carbs
Break	12 oz glass of water, protein powder	Zero carbs
Lunch	12 oz glass of water, Original Tobu Pups, fresh salad greens, black olives, tomato (vinegar and oil) one cup black coffee or tea 12 oz glass of water	Original Tobu Pups—3 links— 6 grams carbs 5 black olives—1.2 grams carbs 1 cup of salad greens— 2 grams carbs
Break	12 oz glass of water, protein powder	Zero carbs
Supper	12 oz glass of water, asparagus spears with melted Soyco Foods Rice Shreds Cheddar Flavor, fresh green salad (vinegar and oil) 12 oz glass of water, tea	8 asparagus spears— 4.4 grams carbs Soyco Foods Rice Shreds Cheddar Flavor—30 gram portion—1 gram carbs 1 cup of salad greens— 2 grams carbs
Day Twenty One	Before bed 12 oz glass of water, if you wake up in the night, drink 12 oz glass of water	Total carbohydrates = less than 30 grams carbs

Day Twenty Two	Vegetarian Menu Eat as much protein as you want! SUBSTITUTE any PROTEIN with a Protein Liberal Vegetarians may add dairy products such as cheese, cream, eggs, or any sea food, fish, or fowl and eat as much as you want!	Carbohydrate Grams Just Limit your Carbohydrates to 30 grams per day!
breakfast	at wake up—12 oz. glass of water, grapefruit, protein powder, one cup black coffee or tea, 12 oz glass of water, vitamins	Half grapefruit— 10.3 grams carbs
Break	12 oz glass of water, protein powder	zero carbohydrates
Lunch	12 oz glass of water, Sunergia Soy-foods More than Tofu Indian Masala, green salad (vinegar and oil) one cup black coffee or tea 12 oz glass of water	Sunergia Soyfoods More than Tofu Indian Masala—2 oz.— 3 grams carbs 1 cup of salad greens— 2 grams carbs
Break	12 oz glass of water, protein powder	zero carbohydrates
Supper	12 oz glass of water, tofu, cabbage, fresh green salad (vinegar and oil) 12 oz glass of water, tea	2 inch cube tofu— 2.9 grams carbs 1 cup cabbage—6.2 grams carbs 1 cup of salad greens— 2 grams carbs
Day Twenty Two	Before bed 12 oz glass of water, if you wake up in the night, drink 12 oz glass of water	Total carbohydrates = less than 30 grams carbs

	Vegetarian Menu	
Day Twenty Three	Eat as much protein as you want! SUBSTITUTE any PROTEIN with a Protein Liberal Vegetarians may add dairy products such as cheese, cream, eggs, or any seafood, fish, or fowl and eat as much as you want!	**Carbohydrate Grams** Just Limit your Carbohydrates to 30 grams per day!
breakfast	at wake up—12 oz. glass of water, protein powder, one cup black coffee or tea, 12 oz glass of water, vitamins	Zero carbs
Break	12 oz glass of water, nuts	3 tablespoons mixed nuts— 7 grams carbs
Lunch	12 oz glass of water, celery and peppers, fresh green salad (vinegar and oil) one cup black coffee or tea 12 oz glass of water	1 stalk of celery— 1.6 grams carbs Quarter cup green peppers—1.8 grams carbs 1 cup of salad greens— 2 grams carbs
Break	12 oz glass of water, nuts	3 tablespoons mixed nuts— 7 grams carbs
Supper	12 oz glass of water, protein powder, cucumbers, mushrooms, peppers fresh green salad (vinegar and oil) 12 oz glass of water, tea	Half cucumber—1.8 grams carbs Half cup mushrooms— 1.6 grams carbs Half pepper—3.2 grams carbs 1 cup of salad greens— 2 grams carbs
Day Twenty Three	Before bed 12 oz glass of water, if you wake up in the night, drink 12 oz glass of water,	Total carbohydrates = less than 30 grams carbs

Day Twenty Four	Vegetarian Menu Eat as much protein as you want! SUBSTITUTE any PROTEIN with a Protein Liberal Vegetarians may add dairy products such as cheese, cream, eggs, or any seafood, fish, or fowl and eat as much as you want!	Carbohydrate Grams Just Limit your Carbohydrates to 30 grams per day!
breakfast	at wake up—12 oz. glass of water, Gimme Lean!, scrambled tofu, one cup black coffee or tea, 12 oz glass of water, vitamins	Gimme Lean! Meatless Sausage Style—2 oz—4 grams carbs 2 inch cube tofu— 2.9 grams carbs
Break	12 oz glass of water, celery	3 stalks celery—4.8 grams carbs
Lunch	12 oz glass of water, Light Life Foney Baloney, fresh green salad (vinegar and oil) one cup black coffee or tea 12 oz glass of water,	Light Life Foney Baloney— 3 slices—2 grams carbs 1 cup of salad greens— 2 grams carbs
Break	12 oz glass of water, protein powder	Zero carbs
Supper	12 oz glass of water, protein powder, collard greens, cabbage coleslaw, fresh green salad (vinegar and oil) 12 oz glass of water, tea	Half cup collard greens— 4.9 grams carbs Half cup cole slaw— 4.25 grams carbs 1 cup of salad greens— 2 grams carbs
Day Twenty Four	Before bed 12 oz glass of water, if you wake up in the night, drink 12 oz glass of water,	Total carbohydrates = less than 30 grams carbs

Day Twenty Five	**Vegetarian Menu** Eat as much protein as you want! SUBSTITUTE any PROTEIN with a Protein Liberal Vegetarians may add dairy products such as cheese, cream, eggs, or any seafood, fish, or fowl and eat as much as you want!	**Carbohydrate Grams** Just Limit your Carbohydrates to 30 grams per day!
breakfast	at wake up—12 oz. glass of water, Lightlife Fakin Bacon, scrambled tofu, one cup black coffee or tea, 12 oz glass of water, vitamins	Lightlife Fakin Bacon Marinated Smokey Tempeh Strips—3 slices—6 grams carbs 2 inch cube of tofu—2.9 carbs
Break	12 oz glass of water, celery	2 stalks celery—3.2 grams carbs 3 tablespoons cream cheese—1.5 grams carbs
Lunch	12 oz glass of water, Smoke and Fire Soy with Sizzle Herb Smoked Tofu, fresh green salad (vinegar and oil) one cup black coffee or tea 12 oz glass of water,	1 cup of salad greens—2 grams carbs Smoke and Fire Soy with Sizzle Herb Smoked Tofu—half cup—2 grams carbs
Break	12 oz glass of water, nuts	One and half tablespoons of mixed nuts—3.5 grams carbs
Supper	12 oz glass of water, protein powder, mushrooms and green beans, fresh green salad (vinegar and oil) 12 oz glass of water, tea	Half cup green beans—3.4 grams carbs Half cup mushrooms—1.6 grams carbs 1 cup of salad greens—2 grams carb
Day Twenty Five	Before bed 12 oz glass of water, if you wake up in the night, drink 12 oz glass of water	Total carbohydrates = less than 30 grams carbs

Day Twenty Six	Vegetarian Menu Eat as much protein as you want! SUBSTITUTE any PROTEIN with a Protein Liberal Vegetarians may add dairy products such as cheese, cream, eggs, or any seafood, fish, or fowl and eat as much as you want!	Carbohydrate Grams Just Limit your Carbohydrates to 30 grams per day!
breakfast	at wake up—12 oz. glass of water, scrambled tofu with celery and peppers, one cup black coffee or tea, 12 oz glass of water, vitamins	2 inch cube of tofu— 2.9 grams carbs 1 stalk celery—1.6 grams carbs Half cup green pepper— 3.6 grams carbs
Break	12-oz glass of water, protein powder	Zero carbs
Lunch	12 oz glass of water, Smoke and Fire Soy with Sizzle Lemon Garlic Smoked Tofu, fresh green salad (vinegar and oil) one cup black coffee or tea 12 oz glass of water	Smoke and Fire Soy with Sizzle Lemon Garlic Smoked Tofu— half cup—3 grams carbs 1 cup of salad greens— 2 grams carbs
Break	12 oz glass of water, celery with Miso Master Organic Red Traditional Soy Paste	2 stalks celery—3.2 grams carbs Miso Master Organic Red Traditional Soy Paste—2 tsp— 4 grams carbs
Supper	12 oz glass of water, protein powder, mushrooms, asparagus spears & melted Soyco Foods Rice Shreds Cheddar Flavor, green salad (vinegar and oil) 12 oz glass of water	4 asparagus spears— 2.2 grams carbs Half cup mushrooms— 1.6 grams carbs Soyco Foods Rice Shreds Cheddar Flavor—30 gram portion —1 grams carb 1 cup of salad greens— 2 grams carbs
Day Twenty Six	Before bed 12 oz glass of water, if you wake up in the night, drink 12 oz glass of water	Total carbohydrates = less than 30 grams carbs

	Vegetarian Menu	Carbohydrate Grams
Day Twenty Seven	Eat as much protein as you want! SUBSTITUTE any PROTEIN with a Protein Liberal Vegetarians may add dairy products such as cheese, cream, eggs, or any seafood, fish, or fowl and eat as much as you want!	Just Limit your Carbohydrates to 30 grams per day!
breakfast	at wake up—12 oz. glass of water, scrambled Smoke and Fire Soy with Sizzle Lemon Garlic Smoked Tofu, one cup black coffee or tea, 12 oz glass of water, vitamins	Smoke and Fire Soy with Sizzle Lemon Garlic Smoked Tofu— half cup—3 grams carbs
Break	12 oz glass of water, nuts	One and half tablespoons of mixed nuts—3.5 grams carbs
Lunch	12 oz glass of water, protein powder, Smart Dogs! and sauerkraut, fresh green salad (vinegar and oil) one cup black coffee or tea 12 oz glass of water	Smart Dogs!—2 links— 10 grams carbs 1 cup of salad greens— 2 grams carbs
Break	12 oz glass of water, celery	3 stalks celery—4.8 grams carbs
Supper	12 oz glass of water, Sunergia Soyfoods More than Tofu Indian Masala, fresh green salad (vinegar and oil) 12 oz glass of water, tea	Sunergia Soyfoods More than Tofu Indian Masala—2 oz.— 3 grams carbs Fresh green salad— 2 grams carbs
Day Twenty Seven	Before bed 12 oz glass of water, if you wake up in the night, drink 12 oz glass of water	Total carbohydrates = less than 30 grams carbs

Day Twenty Eight	**Vegetarian Menu** Eat as much protein as you want! SUBSTITUTE any PROTEIN with a Protein Liberal Vegetarians may add dairy products such as cheese, cream, eggs, or any seafood, fish, or fowl and eat as much as you want!	**Carbohydrate Grams** Just Limit your Carbohydrates to 30 grams per day!
breakfast	at wake up—12 oz. glass of water, scrambled tofu, one cup black coffee or tea 12 oz glass of water, vitamins	2 inch cube tofu—2.9 carbs
Break	12 oz glass of water, protein powder	Zero carbs
Lunch	12 oz glass of water, broccoli, fresh green salad (vinegar and oil), Yves Veggie Cuisine the Good Deli Veggie Ham, one cup black coffee or tea, 12 oz glass of water	Yves Veggie Cuisine the Good Deli Veggie Ham—4 slices—6 grams carbs one cup broccoli—7 grams carbs 1 cup of salad greens—2 grams carbs
Break	12 oz glass of water, celery with nuts	2 stalks celery—3.2 grams carbs One and half tablespoons of mixed nuts—3.5 grams carbs
Supper	12 oz glass of water, protein powder, asparagus with melted Soyco Foods Rice Shreds Cheddar Flavor, fresh green salad (vinegar and oil) 12 oz glass of water, tea	4 spears asparagus—2.2 grams carbs Soyco Foods Rice Shreds Cheddar Flavor—30 gram portion—1 gram carb 1 cup of salad greens—2 grams carbs
Day Twenty Eight	Before bed 12 oz glass of water, if you wake up in the night, drink 12 oz glass of water	Total carbohydrates = around 30 grams carbs

	Vegetarian Menu	Carbohydrate Grams
Day Twenty Nine	Eat as much protein as you want! SUBSTITUTE any PROTEIN with a Protein Liberal Vegetarians may add dairy products such as cheese, cream, eggs, or any seafood, fish, or fowl and eat as much as you want!	**Carbohydrate Grams** Just Limit your Carbohydrates to 30 grams per day!
breakfast	at wake up—12 oz. glass of water, scrambled tofu, one cup black coffee or tea, 12 oz glass of water, vitamins	2 inch cube of tofu— 2.9 grams carbs
Break	12 oz glass of water, protein powder	zero carbs
Lunch	12 oz glass of water, protein powder, peppers, broccoli, fresh green salad (vinegar and oil), one cup black coffee or tea 12 oz glass of water	Half cup cole slaw— 4.25 grams carbs half cup broccoli— 3.5 grams carbs Half cup peppers— 3.6 grams carbs 1 cup of salad greens— 2 grams carbs
Break	12 oz glass of water, celery with nuts	3 stalks celery—4.8 grams carbs One and half tablespoons of mixed nuts—3.5 grams carbs
Supper	12 oz glass of water, protein powder, asparagus, fresh green salad (vinegar and oil) 12 oz glass of water, tea	8 spears asparagus— 4.4 grams carbs 1 cup of salad greens— 2 grams carbs
Day Twenty Nine	Before bed 12 oz glass of water, if you wake up in the night, drink 12 oz glass of water	Total carbohydrates = less than 30 grams carbs

	Vegetarian Menu Eat as much protein as you want! SUBSTITUTE any PROTEIN with a Protein Liberal Vegetarians may add dairy products such as cheese, cream, eggs, or any seafood, fish, or fowl and eat as much as you want!	Carbohydrate Grams Just Limit your Carbohydrates to 30 grams per day!
Day Thirty		
breakfast	at wake up—12 oz. glass of water, Gimme Lean! Meatless sausage style and scrambled tofu, one cup black coffee, or tea, 12 oz glass of water, vitamin	Gimme Lean! Meatless sausage style—2 oz—4 grams carbs 2 inch cube tofu—2.9 grams carbs
Break	12 oz glass of water, protein powder	zero carbs
Lunch	12 oz glass of water, Smart Deli Old World Bologna Style Meatless Slices, cucumbers, tomato, mushrooms fresh green salad (vinegar and oil) one cup black coffee or tea 12 oz glass of water	Smart Deli Old World Bologna Style Meatless Slices—3 slices—2 grams carbs Half cup cucumbers—1.8 grams carbs Half cup mushrooms—1.5 grams carbs Half tomato—2.9 grams carbs 1 cup of salad greens—2 grams carbs
Break	12 oz glass of water, celery	2 stalks celery—3.2 grams carbs
Supper	12 oz glass of water, Smoke and Fire Soy with Sizzle BBQ Smoked Tofu, fresh green salad with mushrooms (vinegar and oil), 12 oz glass of water, tea	Smoke and Fire Soy with Sizzle BBQ Smoked Tofu—half cup—3 grams carbs Half cup mushrooms—1.5 grams carbs 1 cup of salad greens—2 grams carbs
Day Thirty	Before bed 12 oz glass of water, if you wake up in the night, drink 12 oz glass of water	Total carbohydrates = less than 30 grams carbs

30 Days to a Lifestyle Diet

If you are convinced that this diet works, you may wish to continue, so I have a few suggestions for the post 30 Diet Plan. If you are not convinced, go ahead and eat all those sugary delights you crave and notice the return of your weight and unhealthy feeling. It may take a few days, maybe a week or more but your weight will return including any obesity and your health problems will return. You can control your weight, obesity, or health problems with *The Diet*. Here are three suggestions for the future:

First, you should be convinced by now that sugar in all its forms is not for you and should be avoided like the plague.

Also, during the 30 Diet Plan I tried to keep your carbohydrate intake to less than 30 grams a day if you followed my suggestions to prove beyond any doubt that weight is controlled by a high protein diet and that health problems are reduced or even eliminated. After your thirty-day test, you can now decide how many carbohydrates you can tolerate before your weight or your health problems return. You can now experiment with any carbohydrate you want, but I suggest you keep your carbohydrates to less than 50 to 100 grams per day. You may be able to tolerate up to 400 grams a day but you will just have to experiment. If you need help on understanding grams and counting them, the best source is *Protein Power* by Michael R. Eades, M.D. and Mary Dan Eades, M.D. *Sugar Busters*! is an excellent source for this as well. And of course Dr. Atkins has many books on the subject too. You may be able to tolerate even more carbohydrate since each individual is a *diet authority* and can decide what is best. Only you can figure out how many carbohydrates you can tolerate.

Second, if you decide to eliminate sugar in your diet, to control your weight or feel healthier, there are many sources of information on how to live without sugar and you can get many books to help at this online source:

http://rosacea-control.com/html/dietbooks.html

I have picked a long list of books that may be interest to you to choose from at the above url. If you still have doubts that a high protein diet is healthy for you, please read *Protein Power* by Drs. Eades or *Dr. Atkin's New Diet Revolution*. These books are available at the above url for your convenience.

Third, what to do about a well balanced diet after the thirty-day test is not as simple as it may seem. You need to achieve a balance in nutrition without gaining weight or feeling unhealthy and that is the trick. Experimenting with more carbohydrates like grains and fruits can help you decide what is best for you, so you will have to decide how much you can tolerate through trial and error. Eating a sugary dessert may put you back on the road to your previous diet or eventually after eating sugar for a period of time your weight or health problems will return. Taking vitamins as suggested in the chapter on Vitamins and Supplements will help bring about in part a well-balanced nutritional diet. You should at least be happy that you have found a way to control your weight and feel healthier with *The Diet*. You may need additional help from your doctor, other health care professional, or nutritionist with their suggestions on diet. Joining the Diet Users Support Group at yahoo groups is a great way to discuss the three suggestions in these chapters and a way to keep up with the latest information from users of *The Diet*. Many have modified eating and drinking with each individual life style and are happy to offer advice. After all this is a group of *diet authorities*! You may have advice to share. How to join this group is discussed in another chapter. The most important point of *The Diet* is that you have learned to control your weight and feel healthier with your diet.

You may join by copying and pasting this url into your browser:

http://groups.yahoo.com/group/the-diet-support-group

The next chapter gives you information about The *Diet* Users Support Group with some frequently asked questions. This group is an email support group that has two things in common—we all have this book and we want to talk about it. Hopefully it will motivate you to either join the group discussion or at least be a member and read what others are posting. Why not go to the group site and read the posts since they are public knowledge

Diet Users Support Group

How to join: go to this url: http://groups.yahoo.com/group/the-diet-support-group

In the top right corner, click on 'JOIN THIS GROUP'

Set up a yahoo id and password account that gives you an email account with yahoo. **REMEMBER your yahoo id and password. Write it down**.

You can have all group email go to this yahoo email account you register or you have all group email forwarded to your current email account.

Complete the registration form and click on "Submit This Form."

Note: The Yahoo! ID you choose must be unique. It does not need to match your email address.

To join/subscribe to The Diet Support Group via email:

1. Send a blank email to:

the-diet-support-group@yahoogroups.com

2. You will receive a subscription confirmation message. Just reply to this message and your subscription will be complete.

Note: The Diet Support Group is restricted, meaning that the owner or a moderator approves all requests to join. Joining a restricted group sends a message to the owner, who will notify you with an automatically generated email asking you verify you have the book. You should respond to the owner or a moderator that you have the book. Once approved, you will be able to post messages to the group. The exception is if you received an invitation to join, you are pre-approved since your email address is already known and you will not be invited unless someone knows you have the book.

3. You should receive an email confirming your registration. Be sure to record your Yahoo! ID and password. You will need these to sign into Yahoo! Groups.

You may have some questions like these:

What is Yahoo! Groups?

* How much does it cost?
* How do I register?
* How do I start a group?
* How do I transfer my email list to Yahoo! Groups?
* How do I join a group?

* How do I verify my email address?
* How do I unsubscribe from a group?
* Where can I send abuse complaints?
* What is the spam policy in Yahoo! Groups? How do I avoid spam?
* Is it possible for a spammer to gather email addresses from Yahoo! Groups?
* Why am I getting a sign-in error about cookies?

These questions are answered at this url:

http://help.yahoo.com/help/groups/

Setting up your account

Note: You must be signed in with a registered yahoo id and password to use the following features.

* My Preferences allows you to make changes to your account and change your personal preferences. Go here to add email addresses to your account or to verify addresses you've added.
Some questions you may have are answered at the following url:
http://help.yahoo.com/help/us/groups/mypreferences/

* The My Groups page is an easy way to manage your groups and subscription settings.

Some questions you may have are answered at the following url:
http://help.yahoo.com/help/us/groups/mygroups/

* Click on the Account Info link near the top-right corner to change your Yahoo! account and profile information.

These features are always on the top of the group site

How do I verify my email address?
In order to use an email address for Yahoo! Groups, the address must be verified. The easiest way to set up your account is to use the Membership Wizard. The wizard will show all of the email addresses you currently have available for use in Yahoo! Groups. Any unverified addresses will be listed at the bottom of the second page. Next to the address will be a "Verify" link. Click on the link to generate a verification email that will be sent to you at that address. Follow the instructions contained in the email to complete the process.
If the email address you wish to use is not listed, click on the Add new email address link.

Common Member Questions

* What are the options for each of my group subscriptions?
* How can I post a message to a group?
* How long does it take for messages to get delivered to the group?
* Why hasn't a message I sent to the group appeared on the web site?
* How can I put message delivery on hold while I'm away and unable to check email?
* Can I post messages from the web site? Can I post from more than one email address?
* Why did I stop receiving email from my group?
* How do I reactivate my Yahoo! Groups account?

The answers to the above questions are found at:
http://help.yahoo.com/help/us/groups/messages

How do I add a new email address to my Yahoo! Groups account?

Answer found at this url:
http://help.yahoo.com/help/us/groups/mypreferences/mypreferences-07.html

How do I unsubscribe from the group?
Answer found at this url:
http://help.yahoo.com/help/us/groups/groups-32.html

What are the options for each of my group subscriptions?
You have these options for your message delivery for each group:

* Individual Emails
Messages are delivered one at a time to your email inbox. This is the best option if you want to keep up on the latest posts immediately. Email attachments, if included in a message and allowed by your moderator, will be sent directly to you.

* Daily Digest
Messages are delivered in batches of 25 or daily, whichever comes sooner. This is the best option if you want to receive fewer mail messages and don't need up-to-the minute posts in your inbox. Email attachments are not available in digests.

* Only Special Announcements
This means you will receive email messages only when the group moderator posts a "Special Announcement" message. This is a good option if you want to pass on day-to-day discussion for very busy groups but do want to receive important updates from the group moderator. Keep in mind that usage by each moderator will vary. (The moderator may choose to never use this feature, in which case you would never receive email messages, or may choose to use it frequently.)

*No Mail/Web Only
This option puts email message delivery on hold, for example, while you are on vacation. If message archives are available, this option also permits you to read messages at the Yahoo! Groups web site. Note that message archive options are determined by each moderator/owner, and that some groups have no web message archives.
To set any of these options, go to My Groups and choose from the drop-down list of message delivery options for your group.

I suggest you select DIGEST since that is my preference. Try it, you'll like it.

If you have any questions, I will try to answer them if you send an email to the group owner.

Glycemic Index

The Diet uses the carbohydrate gram as the measure to determine total carbohydrate consumption for the day. Many have known about the glycemic index and have asked me about it, but since food labels only carry the carbohydrate gram content, it is difficult to use the glycemic index as a measure when purchasing food. However, according to the Sydney University Glycemic Index Research Service (SUGiRS),

"Consumers across Australia and North America will soon know all about the glycemic index of foods via the new GI symbol on food packages. The GI symbol will appear on a range of foods that have been GI tested by an accredited testing laboratory. All of them will have been tested in 8–10 subjects using standardized methods. The actual GI will appear near the nutrition panel, along with a brief explanation."

We will look to see if this symbol appears on nutrition labels and this may be very helpful to users of *The Diet* to control their weight or feel healthier. Future editions of *The Diet* may cover the glycemic index, but until the GI actually appears on nutrition labels, the carbohydrate gram content is the best source of information for now. More information on this can be found at this url:

http://www.glycemicindex.com/gi_symbl.htm

Sugar Busters! uses the glycemic index and you will find out more useful information.

About the Author

Brady Barrows (b.1950 in Boulder, Colorado) was raised in Texas by his grandparents until age sixteen when he moved to California to live with his father and step-mother, also writers. He graduated from University High School, Los Angeles, California in 1968 and attended Santa Monica College in Santa Monica, California. In 1971 he moved to New Mexico and lived in the Jemez Mountains and became a hippie meeting his wife Betty whom he married. A son, Jeremy, came along in 1973 which by this time the family became Jehovah's Witnesses. In 1994, he joined his wife as a full-time minister of Jehovah's Witnesses and volunteered to do construction work for the Watchtower Bible and Tract Society, Patterson Educational Center, Patterson, New York for six months. Both decided to stay on the East Coast, moving to Great Barrington, Massachusetts where they both have lived since. Brady was diagnosed with rosacea in his thirties in New Mexico and began writing the *Rosacea Diet* in 1999. It was published by iUniverse in 2002. With the success of his first book he wrote *The Diet* for a much larger audience in 2003 published also by iUniverse. Both are still full-time ministers planning on moving west in 2004 to an undisclosed spot in the middle of the Pacific Ocean on one of the Sandwich Islands. Aloha.

Index

0-595-28996-7

www.ingramcontent.com/pod-product-compliance
Lightning Source LLC
Chambersburg PA
CBHW061258280526
45784CB00002B/807